LIFE
AT
RISK

LIFE

Richard D. Land
& Louis A. Moore

EDITORS

AT

RISK

THE CRISES IN MEDICAL ETHICS

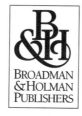

BROADMAN
&HOLMAN
PUBLISHERS

Nashville, Tennessee

© 1995
by the Southern Baptist Christian Life Commission
All rights reserved
Printed in the United States of America

Editing and design by Christian Life Commission Staff
Published by Broadman & Holman Publishers
Nashville, Tennessee

4262-65
0-8054-6265-1

Dewey Decimal Classification: 174
Subject Heading: Medical Ethics
Library of Congress Card Catalog Number: 94-42206

Library of Congress Cataloging-in-Publication Data
Life at risk : the crises in medical ethics / edited by Louis
A. Moore and Richard D. Land.
    p. cm.
    Includes bibliographical references.
    ISBN 0-8054-6265-1
    1. Medical ethics. 2. Christian ethics—Baptist authors.
I. Moore, Louis, 1946– . II. Land, Richard D.
R725.56.L54   1995
174'.2—dc20   94-42206
                                               CIP

Contents

Introduction

I

Crisis at the Beginning

II

Human Genetics

III

Crisis at the End of Life

IV

V

Introduction

By Richard D. Land and Louis A. Moore

This volume originated from the 26th Annual Seminar of the Southern Baptist Christian Life Commission, held in Nashville, Tennessee, in March 1993. The Christian Life Commission staff designed the seminar, entitled "Life at Risk: The Crises in Medical Ethics" to contribute to the ongoing discussion among Southern Baptists about current issues in medicine and medical research today.

The seminar was designed to address such issues as: What is the Humane Genome Project and what are its implications for Christians today? How should Christians respond to the growing "assisted suicide" and euthanasia debate? What does the Bible have to say about the various medical issues? What will be the shape of bioethics in the Third Millennium?

We were mindful that we held the seminar during a time when almost every one of the issues was changing rapidly. For instance, "Dr. Death," also known as Jack Kervokian, was making headlines almost daily even as we met, as he thumbed his nose at the legal/judicial system which was trying to understand his clever maneuvering regarding assisted suicides. But we were also eager to design a seminar that answered questions that extended far beyond 1993 and well into the next century. As medicine changes, so must our understanding of the ethical and moral questions such changes will pose.

This book is divided into five sections, each reflecting the array of issues we must confront. Section 1 is entitled "Crisis at the Beginning" and focuses on life in the womb, starting with conception. Timothy George's outstanding chapter on "Southern Baptists Heritage of Life" details the long and complicated history of Southern Baptists on this issue.

The second section focuses on the Human Genome Project itself. Francis Collins, a Southern Baptist who heads this monumental and important project, which some liken in importance to the Manhattan Project which produced the first atomic bomb, carefully presents a complete description of the significance of all humans because of this project. C. Ben Mitchell, consultant for biomedical and life issues for the Christian Life Commission, wrote a detailed description of the ethical and moral issues the Human Genome Project raises.

The third section focuses on the end-of-life issues. "How do we die?" has become a popular and troubling subject for many Americans today. On the one hand, medical science has the capability to keep people breathing almost for an indefinite period of time, and at the same time others are arguing, even practicing, passive and active forms of euthanasia. Gary Crum, David Biebel and Mark Coppenger all answer the most important questions posed in this debate.

The fourth section offers insight into how Christians can and must respond to this medical revolution. We cannot sit idly by as science rewrites what it means to live and to die. The Bible has much to say about these issues and must not be forgotten in the tidal wave of new scientific advances.

The book closes with an overview that ties all the issues, from the beginning of life to the ending of life together in the important reminder: "We must not fail" by Richard D. Land, executive director of the Southern Baptist Christian Life Commission.

Our hope and desire is that this book will stimulate thinking about these issues—perhaps even become a resource for study by groups of Christians concerned about—maybe even confused about—all the changes that are sweeping our lives.

This book is the third in a series by Broadman & Holman focusing on ethical and moral issues that Southern Baptists must and are confronting today. The first book, which we edited, was entitled *The Earth Is the Lord's*. It detailed how Christians must respond to the growing environmental crisis. The second book, which we also edited, was entitled *Citizen Christians*. It offered insight for how and why Christians must become involved in political issues today.

Our world is changing rapidly, and the issues confronting Christians are changing rapidly, too. We must stay on top of current trends and respond with the ageless message of the prophets of old and the Savior by whose sacrifice on the cross and resurrection from the dead gives us assurance of eternal salvation beyond the medical technologies of this world.

Richard D. Land

Louis A. Moore

Editors

Contributors

Chapter 1. James T. Draper Jr., is president of the Baptist Sunday School Board in Nashville, Tenn., and a former president of the Southern Baptist Convention. He received his B.A. from Baylor University and his M.Div. from Southwestern Baptist Theological Seminary.

Chapter 2. Diane Nutwell Irving is assistant professor of philosophy and bioethics at DeSales School of Theology in Washington, D.C. She received her B.A. degree from Dunbarton College of the Holy Cross, her M.A. and her Ph.D. from Georgetown University in Washington, D.C.

Chapter 3. Carol N. Everett is a pro-life seminar speaker and author who heads Life Network based in Dallas.

Chapter 4. J.C. Willke is president of the International Right to Life Federation and the nationwide Life Issues Institute. A physician, Willke is also past president of the National Right to Life Committee.

Chapter 5. Timothy George is dean of the Beeson Divinity School at Samford University in Birmingham. He is a graduate of the University of Tennessee at Chattanooga, Harvard Divinity School and Harvard University.

Chapter 6. Francis Collins is head of the Human Genome Project. He holds degrees from the University of Virginia, Yale University and the University of North Carolina School of Medicine.

Chapter 7. C. Ben Mitchell is consultant for biomedical and life issues for the Southern Baptist Christian Life Commission. He is a graduate of Mississippi State University and received his M.Div. degree from Southwestern Baptist Theological Seminary. He is currently completing his Ph.D. in philosophy with concentration in medical ethics at the University of Tennessee in Knoxville.

Chapter 8. Kurt P. Wise is assistant professor of science and director of origins research at Bryan College in Dayton, Tenn. He received his bachelor's degree from the University of Chicago and his master's and Ph.D. degrees from Harvard University.

Chapter 9. Thomas Elkins is professor and chairman of the department of obstetrics and gynecology at Louisiana State University Medical School in New Orleans. He received his bachelor's degree from Baylor University and his doctor of medicine from Baylor College of Medicine. He also received a master's degree in religion from Harding University.

Chapter 10. Gary E. Crum is deputy director of policy for the Ohio Department of Health and a former associate professor in the

School of Health Service Management and Policy at George Washington University. He has received degrees from William and Mary College, University of Kentucky, Columbia University and George Washington University.

Chapter 11. David B. Biebel is director of communications for the Christian Medical & Dental Society. He received degrees from Gordon College and Gordon Conwell Theological Seminary.

Chapter 12. Mark Coppenger is vice president for convention relations of the Southern Baptist Convention's Executive Committee. He has received degrees from Ouachita Baptist University, Southwestern Baptist Theological Seminary and Vanderbilt University.

Chapter 13. Thomas R. Harris is chairman of the department of biomedical engineering, director of the division of biomedical engineering and computing and professor of medicine at Vanderbilt University. He holds degrees from Texas A&M University, Tulane University and Vanderbilt University.

Chapters 14 and 15. John MacArthur is pastor of Grace Community Church in Sun Valley, Calif., president of The Master's College, a popular radio preacher and a noted author.

Chapter 16. Franklin E. Payne, Jr., is an associate professor in the department of family medicine and school of medicine at the Medical College of Georgia. He is a graduate of Mercer University and the Medical College of Georgia.

Chapter 17. Joe S. McIlhaney Jr., is a medical doctor, specializing in obstetrical/gynecological care and a noted author on sexuality and reproductive issues. A graduate of Baylor College of Medicine, he established the Medical Institute for Sexual Health, a nonprofit organization.

Chapter 18. Nigel M. de S. Cameron is associate dean of the academic doctoral programs and chair of the department of systematic theology at Trinity Evangelical Divinity School. He has received degrees from Emmanuel College at Cambridge University and from New College at the University of Edinburgh.

Chapter 19. Richard D. Land is executive director of the Southern Baptist Christian Life Commission in Nashville, Tennessee. He holds a B.A. degree from Princeton University, a Th.M. degree from New Orleans Baptist Theological Seminary, and the D.Phil. from Oxford University.

Co-editor Louis A. Moore is an associate vice president at the Foreign Mission Board. Until December 1, 1994 he was director of media and products for the SBC Christian Life Commission. He received his B.A. from Baylor University and his M.Div. from Southern Baptist Theological Seminary.

Preface

Medical science is changing so rapidly these days that it is difficult for many people, including Christians, to keep up with the pace. Surgeries and medical procedures that were once the fodder for science fiction novels are becoming more and more commonplace.

Within a decade, science will have mapped the entire human genome and is already embarked on a once unfathomable quest to wipe out more than 5,000 diseases that find their origin in an individual's genetic code. Each year the average age of Americans expands, and some scientists foresee a lifespan approaching 200 years beginning sometime during the 21st Century.

These changes raise innumerable ethical and moral concerns that few individuals are prepared to handle. Today, the world is confronted with complicated issues such as biogenetic engineering, euthanasia and the harvesting of human tissue.

We compiled this book to stimulate Christian thinking about pressing needs in understanding this rapid scientific and medical development. Throughout the world today, millions of people want to welcome these new advancements, but they also puzzle over the implications of what all of it means for them personally and for their friends and family members. Our own country is leading the world with these discoveries.

This book originated in discussions surrounding the Southern Baptist Christian Life Commission's 26th Annual Seminar in Nashville, Tennessee, in March 1993. It grew out of a belief both at the Christian Life Commission and Broadman Press that serious Christians want to know more about the issues contained on these pages.

Special thanks go to Edith Wilson, the CLC's editorial assistant, and Lee Holloway, who painstakingly checked the manuscripts for accuracy, and to Richard P. "Bucky" Rosenbaum of Broadman & Holman for their guidance throughout the project.

We pray that God will use this book to help enlighten Southern Baptists as well as non-Southern Baptists about the proper biblical response to the multiple medical-ethical issues today.

Richard D. Land
Louis A. Moore
Editors

PART I
Crisis at the Beginning

Crisis Throughout Life

By James T. Draper

At the Beginning of Life (Ps. 139:13-16a)

The word *crisis* has almost lost its meaning today because it is so overused. Every problem seems to be a "crisis." We have the "health-care crisis," the "housing crisis," the "unemployment crisis," the "environmental crisis," the "budget crisis," the "economic crisis," and the "homeless crisis," plus a host of local and personal as well as international "crises."

According to the dictionary, "crisis" means a critical moment, a crucial turning point. We are entirely justified in using that term in connection with the sanctity of life issues in the United States. This is a genuine crisis of monumental proportions. Despite all efforts, we continue to kill at least 1.6 million children each year in this country. The total now is approaching thirty million since *Roe v. Wade* in 1973. We have to wonder how long the Lord will allow this to continue without some severe judgment.

The sanctity of life principle encompasses many issues other than abortion—euthanasia, genetic engineering, fetal tissue experimentation, *in vitro* fertilization, artificial insemination, surrogate motherhood, etc. This is a vast field and one with many ethical and spiritual land mines to negotiate.

Developments in genetics have made reproduction through sexual intercourse only one of several alternatives. *In vitro* fertilization and genetic screening for diseases and abnormalities may result in people going to a hospital to have embryos screened so they can select a baby completely as they want it—sex, normal intelligence, size, etc. Huge questions confront us in this area. Who will have control? Who will benefit? What is God's will and role in the process of procreation?

The issue of surrogate birthing raises not only legal questions but also moral and social questions. These would include at least the "control" issue, issues of family composition, and issues involving parenthood and the marriage bond. Is it the inalienable right of each couple to have a child?

Genetic screening makes it increasingly possible to identify various genetic traits that predispose people to health problems. Approximately two hundred disorders can now be detected prenatally. Such developments have moral/ethical and deeply spiritual implications for the Christian community. Genetics will cause us to rethink and/or reevaluate the deeply religious and biblical issues of life.

The "crisis" of this whole matter is greatly exacerbated when we realize the amount of information concerning genetics more than doubles every two years. Complicating this further is the fact that it is rapidly moving beyond research into commercial applications, and thus broad societal involvement.

As a result of this developing technology, strong and vocal lobbying groups are emerging. These groups will seek to have their views supported and proclaimed by the Christian community through our leaders and our materials. If we do not develop appropriate positions related to these concerns, we will be operating from a defensive or weaker stance in this matter.

As more and more individuals are faced with decisions stemming from the genetic revolution, we must seek to discover what God's Word has to say related to these issues. While all of these areas hold a certain fascination to me, and I would love to develop some discussion on each of them, I want to focus first on the biblical and theological concepts which bear on this "crisis" at the beginning of life.

We must consider and affirm our authority base. As I pointed out in my book, *Authority: The Critical Issue for Southern Baptists,* we have only three possible bases for ultimate authority: (1) human reason, (2) ecclesiastical fiat, or (3) divine revelation.[1] Our great problem in America today arises from the fact that most people are operating from the base of human reason. We will never comprehend the scope of the problem we face until we view it as a basic clash of world views, rather than simply a policy issue or even an isolated ethical issue.

As Christians, we must reaffirm our commitment to divine revelation, i.e. the written Word of God—the Bible—as our ultimate authority base. We listen carefully to what philosophers say, to what secular ethicists say, to what scientists say, to what educators say, to what politicians say, but our ultimate position must depend upon what God says in Scripture!

Frequently we hear the criticism that we are hopelessly inconsistent in our convictions. "You people claim to be 'pro-life,' but while you are dead set against abortion, you support capital punishment. That's hypocritical! Either you are 'pro-life' or you aren't, but you can't have it both ways!"

Such a reaction is not unexpected from those who operate from a base of human reason. If life is sacred, then we should oppose all killing, it would seem to them. But our position must be mandated by Scripture. Scripture opposes abortion (as we shall see), but it authorizes capital punishment. If that seems inconsistent to some, we must remind ourselves and them that Christians are to submit their own reasoning to the authority of Scripture. As Martin Luther said, "My conscience is subject to the Word of God."

Secular humanists today insist that collective human reason provides an adequate consensus for "morality"—"without benefit of clergy," as they like to put it. But the facts of life refute their claim. How do we criticize the Nazi holocaust if that was the "moral consensus" of Germany at the time? If there are no absolutes derived from divine revelation, societies degenerate into either *totalitarianism,* where the dictator determines the rules, or *anarchy,* where every person does what is right in his own eyes (cf. Judg. 21:25). Only the Word of God is eternally immutable and consistent!

Let's focus on the biblical teaching concerning abortion. Does the Bible actually forbid abortion? Virginia Ramey Mollenkott, a self-professed "evangelical feminist," denies that it does. She flatly claims that "nowhere does the Bible prohibit abortion."[2] I assume that Ms. Mollenkott arrived at this rather bizarre conclusion by the use of a biblical concordance. Since she did not find "abortion" listed, she concluded that the Bible doesn't deal with the subject! If one uses this kind of reasoning, we could conclude also that the Bible nowhere forbids the use of crack cocaine, or that it nowhere prohibits insider trading, or whatever. This complete abandonment of classical hermeneutics can hardly be described as "handling the word of truth with precision" (literal rendering of 2 Tim. 2:15).

It is true that the Bible does not use the word *abortion,* nor is there a passage which deals specifically with our modern holocaust. But the Bible does forbid the taking of a human life—except as divinely authorized in the instances of capital punishment and just wars. Therefore, if the Bible considers the preborn child to be a human life, then the Bible forbids abortion.

Before we proceed to the familiar Scripture passages which clearly demonstrate the "humanness" of the preborn child, let me turn to a theological consideration which I believe is crucial. I have rarely seen it mentioned in the abortion debate, and that neglect is puzzling to me. I am not proposing to debate the question of trichotomy vs. dichotomy. It is sufficient for my purpose to point out that I am using both "soul" and "spirit" to refer to the immaterial part of a person, as distinguished from the material body.

Everyone recognizes that the human body proceeds by "natural" generation from the parents. By using the term *natural,* I am not suggesting that God has nothing to do with the process, but that God has ordained that the process occur without an immediate, direct, miraculous, divine intervention. But where does the spirit, or soul, come from? Some theologians have argued that the human spirit is not transmitted by "natural" generation, but is created immediately and miraculously by God and placed in the developing body.

Although most assumed that the "implantation of the spirit" occurred at conception, it was simple enough to hypothesize the "implantation" at viability, or birth, or anywhere else between conception and birth. This rather strange view was thought to be supported by Ecclesiastes 12:7, "Then shall the dust return to the earth as it was: and the spirit shall return unto God who gave it."

This verse does affirm the ultimate separation of the material and immaterial aspects of human beings, and it teaches that, at death, the body goes into the grave and experiences corruption, while the immaterial part of a person, the spirit, goes into the presence of God.

This is the Old Testament counterpart of 2 Corinthians 5:8, "We are confident, I say, and willing rather to be absent from the body, and to be present with the Lord." Although the Ecclesiastes passage affirms that the human spirit comes from God, it *does not* specify *when or how.*

This theory of the "implantation of the spirit" does not harmonize with the biblical doctrines of God and humanity. If we accept the biblical teachings regarding the fall of mankind and the consequent corruption of the race, i.e., the doctrines of original sin and human depravity, we must recognize that the human soul (the immaterial being) is fallen and depraved even as the body is.

Theologians call this the "noetic" (from the Greek *nous,* "mind") effect of the fall. But how did the human soul become depraved if God created it immediately? Did God create a sinful soul to match the sinful body? Unthinkable! God does not create sin—nor does He create sinful beings. His creative acts are *perfect!*

Then, did He place a holy and righteous soul in a fallen, depraved body? This is also unthinkable. We are left, then, with the traditional "Traducian" view, i.e., that the human soul is transmitted, along with the human body, by "natural" generation from the parents. This means, then, that the incipient soul is present at the same time as the beginning of the infant's body. This means that the "fetus" (the operative term in pro-abortion circles today) *has a soul!* It is, thus, a *human being!*

Mere protoplasm doesn't have a soul! It was when God breathed life into the body of Adam that he became a "living soul" (Gen. 2:7). For those who regard Scripture as ultimate authority, this line of theological deduction should be determinative in itself that life begins at conception. This whole idea is further corroborated by David's words in Psalm 51:5, "Behold, I was shapen in iniquity; and in sin did my mother conceive me."

By the way, this concept of the "natural" generation of the soul will give us a basis to make decisions concerning many of the other crises at the beginning of life.

There is much more biblical evidence, of course. The Hebrew word *yeled,* used routinely in the Old Testament for children, is used of the preborn child in Exodus 21:22, "If men strive, and hurt a woman with child, so that her fruit (*yeled*) depart from her. . . ." The "fruit of the womb" is described as children. (I will have more to say about this verse in a different connection.)

The Greek word *brephos* is used in Acts 7:19 to refer to the killing of the children at Pharaoh's command. It is used in Luke 1:41 to refer to John the Baptist while he was still in the womb, "It came to pass, that, when Elisabeth heard the salutation of Mary, the babe (*brephos*) leaped in her womb. . . ." Elisabeth recounts the incident in verse 44, again using *brephos* to refer to the preborn John. Added to this passage is the statement that John the Baptist was filled with the Holy Spirit while still in the womb (Luke 1:15). The Holy Spirit fills (controls) persons—not protoplasm.

Paul testifies that he was set apart and called by God before he was born, "But when it pleased God, who separated me from my mother's womb, and called me by his grace. . ." (Gal. 1:15).

Jeremiah was appointed a prophet to the nations while still in his mother's womb, "Then the word of the Lord came to me, saying, Before I formed thee in the belly I knew thee; and before thou camest forth out of the womb I sanctified thee, and I ordained thee a prophet unto the nations" (Jer. 1:4-5). Isaiah gives a similar testimony, "The Lord hath called me from the womb; from the bowels of my mother hath he made mention of my name" (Isa. 49:1). Job said, "Let the day perish wherein I was born, and the night in which it was said, There is a man child (Hebrew *gaber*) conceived" (Job 3:3). The word *gaber* is frequently used in the Old Testament to mean "man," "male," "boy," or "husband" (cf. Pss. 34:8; 52:7; 94:12). Notice that it was said that a man (or boy) is conceived—not a fetus! The angel of the Lord told Samson's mother that her son would be a Nazarite "from the womb to the day of his death" (Judg. 13:7).

Psalm 139:13-16 is one of the most detailed and explicit passages in all of Scripture concerning God's creative work in the womb. "Reins" (KJV) refers to man's internal organs. "Possessed" means formed or created. "Covered" is literally "knit together." Thus, verse 13 literally reads, "For you have formed (or created) my internal organs; you have knit me together in my mother's womb."

Verse 14 is a beautiful expression of the awe David experienced when contemplating his own creation. (Note that even though we have spoken of "natural" generation, we have used quotation marks to recognize that the hand of God is ultimately involved; parents are simply given the blessed privilege of being instruments of God's creation.)

The "lowest parts of the earth" (v. 15), in context, almost certainly refers metaphorically to the darkness of the womb, although some have suggested Adam's creation from the dust of the earth, or the earth as lower than heaven.

"Curiously wrought" means "intricately made." When we read this beautiful and inspired account of God's work in fashioning the child in the womb, how utterly revolting and sickening becomes the idea of disrupting that divine work by the intrusion of suction devices, poisons, or sharp instruments!

Even though "pro-abortion evangelicals" (An oxymoron if I ever saw one!) continue to suggest that the Bible nowhere forbids abortion, in spite of the massive evidence to the contrary, we need to inquire as to whether they profess to find any Scriptures which support abortion. There is at least one—Numbers 5:11-31, as translated in the New English Bible, and as cited in a tract published by Episcopalians for Religious Freedom, "A Pro Choice Bible Study."[3]

> When a married woman . . . is unfaithful to her husband, and has sexual intercourse with another man . . . and the crime is undetected . . . but when . . . a fit of jealousy comes over the husband which causes him to suspect his wife . . . the husband shall bring his wife to the priest . . . . He (the priest) shall take clean water in an earthenware vessel, and shall take dust from the floor of the Tabernacle and add it to the water. He shall set the woman before the Lord, uncover her head . . . shall . . . put the woman on oath and say to her, '. . . may the Lord make an example of you . . . by bringing upon you *miscarriage and untimely birth* [abortion]; and this water that brings out the truth shall enter your body, bringing upon you *miscarriage and untimely birth.*' The woman shall respond, 'Amen, Amen.' . . . After this he shall make the woman drink the water. If she has . . . been unfaithful to her husband then when the priest makes her drink the water that brings out the truth . . . she will suffer a *miscarriage or untimely birth.* . . . But if the woman has not let herself become defiled and is pure . . . she will bear her child." [Italics added.]

The author of the tract thus concludes that "a planned abortion" is in the Bible as part of God's law given to Moses. Here we presumably have the consent of the parents, plus that of a holy man, to cause an abortion.

In using this passage as the best (only?) biblical passage to be found which might conceivably justify abortion, the pro-abortion religionists demonstrate their desperation. Consider the following points:

1. I am surprised that a group which makes so much of a "woman's right to choose" would select this passage. I would rather expect them to cite this passage as an example of "sexual harassment" in the "ancient Israelite patriarchy."

2. Even if this did refer to a type of "abortion" (which it does not, as we will see), the "abortion" is a miraculous work of God, and is not the work of the parents or the priest. This would thus be totally unlike our modern abortion industry.

3. Most important, the *New English Bible* is inaccurate here. The "miscarriage and untimely birth" should read "making the thigh to shrivel and the abdomen to swell" (see all standard translations). The woman is not pregnant! The sense is that an adulter-

ous woman, so discovered, will find her sexual organs useless—thus, she will be unable to bear children. The passage has absolutely nothing to do with the abortion question!

One other passage, Exodus 21:22-25, is worthy of note :

> If men strive, and hurt a woman with child, so that her fruit depart from her, and yet no mischief follow: he shall be surely punished, according as the woman's husband will lay upon him; and he shall pay as the judge determines. And if any mischief follow, then thou shalt give life for life, Eye for eye, tooth for tooth, hand for hand, foot for foot, Burning for burning, wound for wound, stripe for stripe.

The argument here is not that abortion is justified, but that the fetus is apparently of lesser value than a human life, for the penalty for killing a pregnant woman is death—while the penalty for the death of the fetus is only a fine.[4] But note the following points:

1. Even if the passage is so interpreted, the preborn child is considered of worth, the destroyer of such a preborn child is liable for damages, and there is no mandate for intentional killing of the preborn child.

2. There is considerable doubt as to the legitimacy of this interpretation. A host of commentators, correctly, I believe, take the passage to mean that the mother and the preborn child are of equal value. "Mischief" would then mean the death of either the mother or her child. If the accident results in a premature birth, but the mother and child both survive—then a fine is in order. If either should die, however, the death penalty is appropriate. This passage underscores the value and worth God places upon the preborn child.

From Scripture let me draw some conclusions that can help us build a foundation for decisions and action. All understanding of God in Scripture ultimately comes from the revelation that He is our Creator. Confession of God as Creator means He created me. If He created me, He knows everything about me. The emphasis here is not simply that God knows everything in general, that He is omniscient, but that He knows everything about us personally. He knows our thoughts and motivations, our words and deeds. The emphasis is upon God's knowledge as it relates to us.

David's point is not that God is everywhere present—always and at the same time—but that everywhere we turn, we are confronted by the God who knows us thoroughly.

God's intense knowledge of me leads to my intense gratitude to Him for life, a life that can only be explained in terms used for God's acts of salvation history—wonderful, awesome. My life is almost seen as one part of His salvation history. It is important for us to realize that God will not leave the work of His own hands (Ps. 138:8) either to chance or to ultimate extinction.

There can be little doubt, then, as to the scriptural mandate for the protection of the preborn child. Our abortion scandal is driven by forces quite alien to Scripture and the historic Christian faith. The understanding of this fact and a close study of Scripture can guide us through this immense crisis at the beginning of life.

At the End of Life (Ps. 139:16b)

The growing disregard for life is invading every aspect of our society. It began with abortion on demand. It continued with infanticide. Now it appears as if euthanasia will become an accepted part of our society. It is already a major concern in the Netherlands. Between 6,000 and 10,000 people die by euthanasia every year in that country, even though active euthanasia is still a criminal offense.[5]

Without a doubt, unless some other factor is injected into the situation, the moral decline in this country will continue unabated. Future generations will practice evils which we today abhor. The "other factor" that must be injected into this entire discussion is a Christian presence and Christian opposition to evil in society. Nowhere is our need to be salt and light more evident than here.

The issues at the end of life are crucial. Some basic under-standings are necessary if we are to properly address these issues. Robert Rakestraw wrote in the *Journal of the Evangelical Theological Society,* September 1992, a most helpful article dealing with some of these problems. In that article he spoke of the mean-ing of the "image of God." He said,

> To be in the 'image of God' means that we exist as the representatives of God on earth, with certain God-given and God-like qualities and capacities, so that we may experience vital relationships with God and others and so that we may exercise dominion over the earth.... Given this understanding of the image concept, we may now attempt a definition of the term 'person.' A human person is a unique individual, made as God's image, known and cared for by God at every stage of life, with the actual ability or potential to be aware of oneself and to relate in some way to one's environment, to other

human beings, and to God. The earthly life of a person thus begins at conception and ends when this ability or potential ceases.[6]

The real question for the Christian is, when does death occur? At what point is a person dead? Medically, there are various opinions about this. As Christians we must consider God's revelation in His Word in formulating ethical judgments about such matters.

There are many forces moving in this arena today. Dr. Jack Kervorkian advocates "assisted suicides" for patients who are terminally ill or who choose to end their lives. At the other end of the spectrum is the case of Nancy Cruzan, the first "right-to-die" case to reach the U.S. Supreme Court. Critically injured in a car accident, her brain received no oxygen for fourteen minutes. She lay in a comatose condition for approximately eight years, with the expectation of living thirty or forty years in that state without some action. The parents were eventually authorized to remove the feeding tube, and her life came to an end on December 26, 1990.

The Christian community split in its opinion of this case. Joseph Foreman, a founder of Operation Rescue, called Cruzan's death a tragedy. "I think in the next few years you will see an entire industry spring up around putting people to death whom family, friends, and so forth have deemed to be no longer of use to anybody. There will be wings of hospitals devoted to putting people to death like this."[7]

On the other side was Kenneth Schemmer, an Orange County, California, surgeon, and member of First Evangelical Free Church of Fullerton. He held that Cruzan should be allowed to die. "Nancy actually died on January 11, 1983, of anoxia" as the result of her car accident, which produced cardiorespiratory arrest. Because Nancy's cerebral cortex—the seat of consciousness, reasoning, value decisions, and everything else we associate with personality—was so severely damaged that it no longer functioned, only her living "animal" body remained. Her "mammalian body" should be allowed to die.[8]

Clearly the issue is complicated and requires our best understanding to formulate a proper Christian response. An illustration of the complexity of these matters is the case of Jacqueline Cole. On March 29, 1986, she collapsed with a massive hemorrhage in the brain. Virtually no hope was held for her recovery. Doctors concluded that if she did survive she would be in a permanently vegetative state. After much prayer, her preacher husband and family determined that it would be best to remove her from the life support system. However, Judge John Carroll Byrnes declined permission, citing "too brief a time has elapsed," and asking for more legal precedents.

Six days later, on May 15, 1986, Jackie responded to the greeting of an old family friend by opening her eyes. She responded to her husband's stunned question, "Jackie, are you awake?" by nodding, smiling, and returning his kiss. Some of the time the intervention of God reminds us of the inability of finite humans to make life and death decisions.[9]

The direction our society is moving is clearly defined for us. Dr. Peter Singer wrote an article in *Pediatrics,* the official journal of the American Academy of Pediatrics, entitled "Sanctity of Life or Quality of Life?"[10]

> Once the religious mumbo-jumbo surrounding the term "human" has been stripped away, we may continue to see normal members of our species as possessing greater capacities of rationality, self-consciousness, communication, and so on, than members of any other species; but we will not regard as sacrosanct the life of each and every member of our species, no matter how limited his capacity for intelligent or even conscious life may be. If we compare a severely defective human infant with a sub-human animal, a dog or a pig, for example, we will often find the non-human to have superior capacities, both actual and potential, for rationality, self-consciousness, communication and anything else that can plausibly be considered morally significant. . . . Humans who bestow superior value on the lives of all human beings, solely because they are members of our own species, are judging along lines strikingly similar to those used by white racists, merely because they are members of their own race.

Dr. Singer is a philosopher, not a medical doctor, but the fact that the editors of *Pediatrics* would publish such an article is highly significant—and not a little frightening!

Philip Dunne wrote in the January 15, 1990, issue of *Time* magazine: "At the heart of the right-wingers' argument is their lingering hope that, as other generations believed, our species was singled out for a special creation in God's own image."[11]

Note his reference to "right-wingers" and their rather quaint "lingering hope" of creation in God's image!

In a recent textbook on Christian ethics, John and Denise Carmody discuss the question of medical priorities:

Christian ethicists could also do more to spotlight the dangers in considering U.S. problems in isolation from the rest of the world. Though it is true that Americans still do not get optimal health care, compared with the care available in Third World countries American medicine can seem a luxury. So the question arises: How moral is it to concentrate huge resources in areas where health care already is adequate, while the majority of the world suffers grossly inadequate health care? . . . Christian ethicists have to reckon with the question of the morality of expending billions of dollars prolonging the lives of the elderly while allowing the young of the Third World, or of the minority populations of the United States, to go neglected. . . . The more critical the world's health needs, the more closely we approach the catastrophic situation in which triage has to be a fact of life. This notion, developed on the battle field, separates those needing attention into three categories. The principles of separation are, who has the most dire need, and who is most likely to benefit from our limited resources (time, medicine, space)? Those most likely to benefit, and most needing immediate attention, become the top priority. Those offering the least prospect of surviving become the lower priority....
In a broader perspective, children should be the top priority, because restoring children to full health bids to prolong the race for many years.[12]

I use this lengthy quotation to demonstrate the trend of modern thinking away from a "sanctity of life" perspective to a more utilitarian stance. You will note that the elderly do not fare well in this new thinking. Note also the distortion of the concept of triage in this reasoning. Obviously, the military situation is a necessary adjustment to emergency situations. However, even then there is no concept of treating the casualties in the order of their potential importance to the war effort or to humanity.

We have a rising crescendo of voices which questions the moral necessity of preserving every human life, if some egalitarian or utilitarian purpose can better serve the cause of humanism. We need to back off and take a broader view of the entire problem. Our abortion crisis, our increasing infanticide problem, our rapid movement toward euthanasia are symptoms of the larger problem we face—a world-view problem. Our concept of the sanctity of life arises from a Christian world view.

13

The opposing concepts arise from a naturalistic, humanistic, utilitarian world view. We must understand this! About two hundred years ago, beginning with a Scottish geologist named James Hutton, called "the father of uniformitarianism," followed by Charles Lyell in the 1830s with his enormously influential *Principles of Geology,* and leading to Charles Darwin's works in the 1850s through the 1870s, the uniformitarian, evolutionary scheme took shape and quickly began to dominate the natural sciences—and, subsequently, the social sciences as well.

In this view humans are seen as animals—highly advanced animals, to be sure—but still animals. The difference between humans and the "other animals" is one of degree, not of kind. There is no concept of deity, no concept of divine creation, no concept of creation in God's image. Thus, there is nothing corresponding to the biblical concept of the sanctity of human life, because human life is, intrinsically, no more valuable and precious than other forms of animal life, except as the "survival of the fittest" produces greater utilitarian value. When we grasp the evolutionary world view which drives these people, we can begin to understand why a person who favors abortion for convenience would also, logically, find no problem with the various forms of euthanasia.

All of this, of course, has led to unspeakable horrors in this century. Adolf Hitler is an awful example. Sir Arthur Keith summarizes the Third Reich: "The German Fuhrer . . . consciously sought to make the practice of Germany conform to the theory of evolution."[13]

He went on to say: "The leader of Germany is an evolutionist, not only in theory, but, as millions know to their cost, in the rigor of its practice. . . . He regards himself . . . as the incarnation of the will of Germany, the purpose of that will being to guide the evolutionary destiny of its people."[14]

Keith's analysis is corroborated by a reading of *Mein Kampf,* in which Hitler spoke of "lower human types," criticized the Jews for bringing "Negroes into the Rhineland" with the aim of "ruining the white race by the necessarily resulting bastardization," and spoke of "monstrosities halfway between man and ape."[15]

How fundamentally and radically different is all of this from what the Word of God says. Let's review the biblical foundations for the concept of the sanctity of human life.

1. Creation. The Bible teaches that Adam was created directly and immediately by God from the dust of the earth—not from any previously existing form of life. "And the Lord God formed man of the dust of the ground, and breathed into his nostrils the breath of life; and man became a living soul" (Gen. 2:7). In Genesis 2:21-25, we read that God created Eve immediately and miraculously from Adam's side. Subsequently, God designed the creative process which would allow Adam and Eve to participate in the procreation of offspring.

2. In God's Image. Not only were we created directly and miraculously by God, the Bible says we were created in God's image. "And God said, Let us make man in our image, after our likeness: and let them have dominion over the fish of the sea, and over the fowl of the air, and over the cattle, and over all the earth, and over every creeping thing that creepeth upon the earth. So God created man in his own image, in the image of God created he him; male and female created he them" (Gen. 1:26-27).

This image of God dramatically sets humans apart from the animals, among whom Adam found no suitable mate (Gen. 2:20). Humans indeed were to have dominion over the animals! Dr. Singer's bizarre comment about the relative value of dogs, pigs, and human beings is totally foreign to the biblical world view. It is a thoroughly pagan position.

3. In God's Plan. Since humans are created by God in His own image, it is not surprising to learn from Scripture that God has a plan for each individual's life. Psalm 139:16b (NIV) says, "All the days ordained for me were written in your book before one of them came to be." Ephesians 2:10 says, "For we are his workmanship, created in Christ Jesus unto good works, which God hath before ordained that we should walk in them." If God has ordained our life span and has ordained what He wished us to accomplish during that time period (which only He knows), how wicked it is for us to shorten that span (euthanasia) or eliminate it altogether (abortion)! Man is not to play God!

4. God's Special Love. Both the very young and the elderly are singled out in Scripture as special objects of God's love and provision. "Lo, children are an heritage of the Lord: and the fruit of the womb is his reward. As arrows are in the hand of a mighty man; so are children of the youth. Happy is the man that hath his quiver full of them . . ." (Ps. 127:3-5). What a stark contrast to abortion and infanticide!

Passages such as Leviticus 19:32, "Thou shalt rise up before the hoary head, and honour the face of the old man, and fear thy God," show God's special compassion for older people. They are not useless in His sight. How different from the ominous portents of euthanasia in our day!

5. Death and the Fall. Most modern secularists see death as the end of all existence for the life form that experiences it—including man. It is viewed as a natural part of the evolutionary process. The Bible, on the contrary, views death as the direct result of Adam's fall—and thus an enemy of human life. (Cf. 1 Cor. 15:26, where death is described as "the last enemy.")

Since this is the case, death is to be regarded as an unnatural intrusion into God's creation and, thus (logically), to be resisted as long as possible (unless God's will is clearly otherwise). This concept has been a major influence on the medical profession. Physicians, as reflected in the Hippocratic Oath, have been regarded as healers—not killers!

Since the Bible teaches that death brings one ultimately before God for judgment (Heb. 9:27, "It is appointed unto men once to die, but after this the judgment"), it is a serious matter indeed to intentionally shorten a person's life—when an extension might bring that person to salvation! I have thought of this every time I have heard of the latest "assisted suicide" by Dr. Jack Kervorkian. Does this man never consider the awesome responsibility he assumes when he launches a human being into eternity prematurely? His activities point up the difference which must be maintained between "causing a person to die" and "letting a person die." Although some would use the term *euthanasia* to cover both instances, we must insist upon maintaining a clear distinction between the two, reserving the term *euthanasia* for a deliberate act of killing, even though the perpetrators may imagine that such killing is merciful.

The term *euthanasia* comes from the Greek—*eu,* "good"; and *thanatos,* "death"—therefore, literally "good death" or "death with a good end in mind."

It is quite a different thing to "pull the plug" on a brain-dead patient with no hope of recovery from denying a handicapped child life-saving surgery—or even food and water—as in the infamous "Baby Doe" case in Indiana. Once again we see the stark difference between the sanctity of life and the quality of life.

Who indeed is sufficient to determine the suitability of one's "quality of life"? Parents? Other relatives? The state? Is it not obvious that only God should be allowed to make that decision? When human beings begin to make such calls (and ultimately it will likely be the state), we open the door not only to abortion on demand, but widespread infanticide and euthanasia as well. This is not theoretical possibility; this is happening in the United States of America today! What can Christians do?

A People in Crisis (Ps. 139:17-24)

In a few years we will reach the end of this decade, the end of the twentieth century, and the end of the second millennium since Christ. It may well be that the crises which the church faces will prove to be as significant as any in church history.

The crisis which we face in medical ethics seems to be worsening rather rapidly with the inauguration of the current administration in Washington. Note what took place in just a few short weeks after the inauguration of the current administration:

1. The ban on abortion counseling in federally funded clinics was rescinded.

2. The ban on utilization of aborted fetuses for medical research was lifted—renewing the fear of wholesale "harvesting" of preborn children for this purpose.

3. Mr. Clinton moved to legalize the French abortion pill RU-486.

4. The appointment of pro-abortion justices to the Supreme Court became a certainty.

5. The passage of the Freedom of Choice Act, which would take abortion out of the hands of the courts and the state legislatures and would permit no limits on the killing of preborn children became quite possible. It would make *Roe v. Wade* appear almost conservative by comparison.

Add to all of this the high-profile agenda to legitimize homosexuality in America (in the military and elsewhere), the push for "safe sex" education (with furnished condoms) in our schools, the almost certain liberalization in funding policy at the National Endowment for the Arts, the movement toward more and more state control of our children, and Christians in the United States can hardly be blamed for being extremely apprehensive, if not downright discouraged and frustrated.

Popular Christian speakers such as Charles Colson are predicting a "new dark age." Theologians such as Carl F. H. Henry are speaking of an era of "neo-paganism." Conservative politicians such as Pat Buchanan are warning of "a battle for the soul of America."

What are we do to? What are the proper responses for the church in such days?

It is obvious that there is a great gap between biblical beliefs and principles and public policy in the areas we have discussed thus far. It is imperative that we as Christians address that gap and bridge it. The response we make to this crisis may well be our

17

greatest legacy to the world of tomorrow. It is vital that we act biblically, responsibly, and compassionately in this matter.

The truths of Psalm 139 must be foundational for us in these days. God made each of us uniquely and individually. He determined our times and circumstances. He knows all of our thoughts and deeds, even before they occur. He holds all of us accountable to Him for our actions and thoughts. He extends to us the opportunity to turn to Him in loyalty.

> How precious also are thy thoughts unto me, O God! how great is the sum of them! If I should count them, they are more in number than the sand: when I awake, I am still with thee. Surely thou wilt slay the wicked, O God: depart from me therefore, ye bloody men. For they speak against thee wickedly, and thine enemies take thy name in vain. Do not I hate them, O Lord, that hate thee? and am not I grieved with those that rise up against thee? I hate them with perfect hatred: I count them mine enemies. Search me, O God, and know my heart: try me, and know my thoughts: And see if there be any wicked way in me, and lead me in the way everlasting (Ps. 139:17-24).

David's great concern is that nothing in himself would cause God to be offended. He asks for God's examination of his heart and his motives and declares his commitment to following God throughout all his life. That must be our position as we face this challenging age. Our greatest desire must be that we please God! Let me propose some suggestions for Christian action in this day of challenge.

1. Concerning legislating morality. The cliche, "You can't legislate morality," is so commonly heard that even some Christians are taken in by it as though it were an irrefutable axiom of life. But let's look at that statement for a moment. Consider the words of Kerby Anderson:

> Part of the confusion stems from blurring the distinctions between law and human behavior. When a person says, 'You can't legislate morality,' he or she may mean simply that you can't make people good through legislation. In that instance, Christians can agree. The law (whether biblical law or civil law) does not by itself transform human behavior. The Apostle Paul makes that clear in his epistle to the Romans. English jurists for the last few centuries have also agreed that the function of the law is not to make

humans good, but to control criminal behavior. But if
you understand the question in its normal formulation,
then Christians can and should legislate morality.[16]

When you really think about it, there is precious little to legislate except morality! Laws against murder, laws against theft, laws against restraint of trade, are *all* attempts to legislate morality. All criminal law and most of civil law attempts to legislate morality. The question is not *whether* to legislate morality, but *what* morality to legislate.

We pride ourselves in this country on our freedoms—but there are limits. Your right to swing your arm freely stops at my nose! You cannot yell, "Fire!" in a crowded building. Government must legislate the limits of human freedom.

In our present context, this means we must continue to press for laws that will honor the sanctity of human life. Organizations such as the Southern Baptist Christian Life Commission play a strategic role in these matters—in educating politicians, and in keeping us all better informed of the current issues. Even in times of potential discouragement, such as now, we must not relax in this area. Even when we seem to be losing ground on every side, we must not concede the field to our adversaries.

2. Concerning fighting the battle as Christians. For some time now, Christians have attempted to camouflage our concerns under the euphemisms "traditional values" or "family values." Our strategy, I suppose, was to downplay the "Christian" aspect of our values, thinking this would turn some people off, and instead play on the residual decency of the American people, whether professed Christians or not. We hoped for some continuation, at least, of the "Christian consensus" (to use Francis Schaeffer's term) which once held our society together.

I suggest, with considerable sadness, that such a consensus may no longer exist in this country. It is very difficult for those of us who are a little older to come to grips with what has happened, with sickening rapidity, in our land—but we must. Did those of us over fifty think we would live to see the day in the United States of America when we would be killing over 1.6 million preborn children every year? Would we have believed that militant homosexuals would parade openly by the tens of thousands through our city streets demanding their "rights"? Would we have believed the corruption and utter filth now seen on our movie and television screens?

How did all of this happen so quickly? What went wrong? The answer is a theological one. The rapid decline in American morality is in direct proportion to the theological decline in the once great Protestant denominations. As long as our churches were strong, our society was strong. When the churches, one after another, like bowling pins, began to fall to rationalistic, humanistic theological innovations, the nation lost its moral compass. And the only way that our nation can regain its moral bearings is for the church to again become a prophetic voice, rather than a pale reflection of the culture.

It is time we began to talk about *Christian values—biblical values*. Traditions change, "but the word of the Lord endureth for ever" (1 Pet. 1:25). But won't people be "turned off" by such blatant Christian proclamation? Possibly—at first—but we must remember that "the word of God is living and powerful, and sharper than any two-edged sword" (Heb. 4:12, NKJV). Paul tells us of a time "when they will not endure sound doctrine," when "they shall turn away their ears from the truth" (2 Tim. 4:3-4).

What are Christians to do in such times? Be quiet so as not to offend? Paul commands, "Preach the word; be instant in season, out of season; reprove, rebuke, exhort with all longsuffering and doctrine" (2 Tim. 4:2). The organized church of Jesus Christ has become like a trumpet giving an uncertain sound. Is it any wonder that our people are confused and rudderless, like sheep without a shepherd?

3. Concerning the Christian's battle. The Christian life, according to Scripture, is a continuous spiritual battle—in every age and societal context. We are to "war a good warfare" (1 Tim. 1:18), realizing that "the weapons of our warfare are not carnal" (2 Cor. 10:4), but spiritual. We are to "fight the good fight of faith" (1 Tim. 6:12). We are to "put on the whole armour of God" (Eph. 6:11).

It may well be in the Ephesians passage particularly that Christians today will find the means of coping with the deadly serious battle that we face, a battle, Paul tells us, against *spiritual* forces—even though they may present themselves to us in tangible forms. We must have the "whole armour"—not just part of it. An "Achilles' heel" will mean defeat. Let's review briefly the pieces of the armor.

(1) *The girdle (or belt) of truth.* This is experiential, not abstract. It refers to the Christian's sincerity, candor, or openness toward God. No sham, no hypocrisy—the genuine article. The world is sick unto death of religious hypocrites! We will never make much impact on our society until we can demonstrate that our Christianity is real.

(2) *The breastplate of righteousness.* A companion piece of armor. The reference again is to experience, not position. The Christian must be morally pure and upright himself before he can suggest how others ought to live.

(3) *The "combat boots" with the "firm footing" of the gospel of peace.* The primary reference here is to the "peace with God" (Rom. 5:1) which Christians enjoy in salvation; i.e., we cannot engage the enemy in battle unless we are certain that we are in right relationship with God through Jesus Christ.

(4) *The shield of faith.* This is the means whereby the Roman soldier turned away the flaming arrows, and the means by which the Christian turns away all doubts and attacks upon his own faith. We lose many in the battle for the lack of this shield.

(5) *The helmet of salvation.* Note 1 Thessalonians 5:8, "the hope of salvation." This is our certainty of the future in Christ's presence. Regardless of the current state of the battle, we know who ultimately wins! This is why we must not become discouraged. We are on the winning side. "The kingdoms of this world are become the kingdoms of our Lord, and of his Christ; and he shall reign for ever and ever" (Rev. 11:15).

(6) *The sword of the spirit.* Here is our only offensive weapon—the Word of God! As already mentioned, we must use this Word, even when human reason doubts that it will be effective!

4. Concerning the strategy of the battle. It is to be expected that Christians will sometimes differ as to the strategy and tactics in the battle against ungodliness. An example of this is in the matter of Operation Rescue. This group's sincerity, courage, and commitment to the Lord Jesus Christ and to the sanctity of life is unquestioned. However, individuals just as committed and as sincere question the value of their strategy. If the purpose of that strategy is to lessen the number of immediate abortions simply by blocking the doors of abortion clinics, then the effectiveness of the effort must be questioned. If the overriding purpose of the demonstrations is to show the American people, through the extensive media coverage, that abortion is wrong and that there are many who oppose it, then that goal must be evaluated. The polls indicate that such actions harden the pro-abortion people in their stance, and turn uncommitted people away from the pro-life movement—all of this in spite of the noble motives of the people involved.

I am not entering into the question of whether this strategy is correct, but simply pointing out that we must evaluate and prayerfully use good common sense in the battle that is before us, in addition to our zeal and commitment.

5. Concerning prayer. When we mention the need for prayer, there will be no dissenting voice. Of course, we must pray. We all agree. Prayer is essential. Prayer changes things. But I am convinced that evangelicals in this generation talk about prayer more and pray less than any generation in church history.

Take one example. What is the single least-attended meeting at your church? Prayer meeting, of course. Polls show that the average Christian minister prays less than five minutes per day. Most of us are simply not serious about prayer. It is entirely possible that God may be allowing American Christians to move into a situation where prayer becomes an urgent necessity rather than an ecclesiastical formality.

We may be approaching the time when God must move in our midst, or we may face total moral and spiritual collapse. We speak much of the need for revival in our country, but, candidly, much of the talk seems more programmatic than biblical. Many feel that "revival" would be a "neat" addition to our church calendar—perhaps we could schedule it somewhere between Vacation Bible School and Sunday School Promotion Day!

However, except for a few, we don't really have a sense of urgency. How many Southern Baptists are beseeching God daily for a divine visitation in our day—not just as a formal exercise, but out of a sense of desperate need? Let us all be reminded of Proverbs 21:1, "The king's heart is in the hand of the Lord, as the rivers of water: he turneth it whithersoever he will." We may be feeling frustration and discouragement, but God is neither frustrated nor discouraged. He is not defeated.

The oft-quoted 2 Chronicles 7:14 has become almost an evangelical cliché, I am afraid, but let me urge us to listen to it once more—carefully—prayerfully—as though we were hearing it for the first time: "If my people, which are called by my name, shall humble themselves, and pray, and seek my face, and turn from their wicked ways; then will I hear from heaven, and will forgive their sin, and will heal their land."

Furthermore, we must not forget our biblical mandate to be in subjection to and pray for those in authority over us. I sense that many of us are finding this to be more difficult right now than at almost any time of our lives. But the Word of God is clear. Romans 13:1 declares, "Let every soul be subject unto the higher powers. For there is no power but of God: the powers that be are ordained of God." The "powers that be" means the powers currently in office, and when Paul wrote Romans, that meant Nero. Even the most fervent voice among us would likely admit that Nero was worse than any leader we have today!

Not only are we to be in subjection—we are to pray. 1 Timothy 2:1-3 says:

> I exhort therefore, that, first of all, supplications, prayers, intercessions, and giving of thanks, be made for all men; For kings, and for all that are in authority; that we may lead a quiet and peaceable life in all godliness and honesty, For this is good and acceptable in the sight of God our Saviour. . . ." This, of course, does not mean that we must agree with our rulers, nor does it prevent us from working to change their intentions and actions—by all appropriate means. It does mean that we are to honor the offices which they hold and to beseech God in their behalf.

6. Concerning evangelism. We have pointed out that our crisis is a world-view crisis. We will not change many minds regarding the sanctity of life until we change hearts. The Great Commission still stands as the marching orders of the church. It is no coincidence that when people come to faith in Christ, they also begin to change their views about life's great issues. It is not an accident that most pro-lifers are Christians—or that most pro-abortionists and pro-euthanasiasts are unbelievers. The decline in influence of evangelical Christianity in this country in this generation can be traced directly to the fact that there are fewer evangelical Christians (proportionately) now. In other words, our sagging evangelistic efforts have had national, as well as ecclesiastical, ramifications. We need to recapture the vision of the church as a mighty spiritual army, marching across the land, sweeping multitudes into the kingdom of God.

On July 18, 1940, during one of the darkest hours in Britain's history, Winston Churchill rallied his people. He stated that the battle of France was now over, and the battle of Britain was about to begin. On the outcome of the battle, he said, rested the cause of Western civilization.

Listen to his concluding words:

> Let us, therefore, brace ourselves to our duties and so bear ourselves that if the British empire and its commonwealth lasts for a thousand years, men will still say, 'This was their finest hour!'

So let us recommit ourselves to the great verities of the historic Christian faith; let us recommit ourselves to renewed witness; let

23

us "pray and not faint." Let us see what God will do for us, and through us in these days.

And let us remember, as Psalm 139 tells us, the people of life stand for moral integrity, identifying with God's values and not merely human values. People of God place themselves before God's judgment, aware of the mystery of His omnipotence, omniscience, and omnipresence. We invite God to judge, convict, and change us as we seek His leadership through all of life's difficult moral and spiritual decisions. And we confess our renewed loyalty to Him and to the truth of His Word. He is our Creator God, our Sovereign Lord. May we be truly the people of life in this darkened and degenerate age.

Endnotes

[1]James T. Draper, *Authority: The Critical Issue for Southern Baptists* (Old Tappan, N.J.: Fleming H. Revell Company, 1984): 16.

[2]Virginia Ramey Mollenkott, "Reproductive Choice: Basic to Justice for Women," *Christian Scholar's Review* (March 1988): 291.

[3]Cited by Francis J. Beckwith, "A Critical Appraisal of Theological Arguments for Abortion Rights," *Bibliotheca Sacra* (July-September 1991): 346-348.

[4]See, for example, J. Coert Rylaarsdam, "Exodus," in *The Interpreter's Bible,* ed. G. A. Buttrick et. al., 12 vols. (New York: Cokesbury-Abingdon Press, 1951-57): 1:999.

[5]See *Eternity* magazine(March 1988): 46-49.

[6]*Journal of the Evangelical Theological Society,* (September 1992): 400-401.

[7]"A Peaceful Death Ends Fight Over Nancy Cruzan," [Minneapolis] *Star Tribune* (December 27, 1990): 1A, 14A.

[8]K. E. Schemmer, "Nancy Cruzan Is Already Dead," (Loma Linda University Ethics Center) Update 5 (December 1989): 4-5.

[9]*Eternity* Magazine (March 1988): 50.

[10]Cited by John J. Davis, *Evangelical Ethics* (Phillipsburg, N. J.: Presbyterian and Reformed Publishing Company, 1985):169.

[11]Philip Dunne, "Dissent, Dogma and Darwin's Dog," *Time* (January 15, 1990): 84.

[12]John and Denise Carmody, *Christian Ethics* (Englewood Cliffs, N.J., Prentice Hall, 1993): 201-202.

[13]*Evolution and Ethics*, (Putnam's, 1947): 230—cited in *Impact* (February 1987):1.

[14]Ibid.

[15]*Mein Kampf,* Houghton Mifflin, 1943: 286, 295, 325, 402-403, 285, 289 - Ibid.

[16]J. Kerby Anderson, "A Christian Perspective," *Kindred Spirit* (Autumn 1988): 3.

Fetal "Personhood"

By Dianne Nutwell Irving

We find ourselves engulfed in one ethical dilemma after another these days—many brought on by the explosion of medical technology. At times it seems that the "theory" has not had time to catch up with the pace of these rapid changes. We especially, as Christians, find it difficult—and sometimes even downright embarrassing—to seek clarification, or even frame our responses, from our Christian faith's perspective. We must respond. Yet how relevant can our responses possibly be these days, if grounded in our "Christian traditions"? Doubts abound!

Such, frankly, were my anxious thoughts as well, as I prepared to confront the literature on fetal personhood.[1] Fairly convinced initially that "personhood" probably started at about fourteen days, based on my rough survey of the arguments, I settled into sorting out the mile-high stack of articles. Some argued for "immediate personhood," i.e., at fertilization there is present a human being who is necessarily and simultaneously a human person. Some, on the other hand, argued for "delayed personhood," i.e., at some later point during human embryogenesis an embryo or fetus finally becomes either a human being or a human person. These latter embryological events are referred to as the "biological marker events of fetal personhood."

However, I realized fairly quickly that not only was the *philosophy* used in these debates often "a little weird," but more disturbing to me, as a former research chemist and biologist, the *science* used was textbook-incorrect in virtually *all* of the arguments (other than those arguing for "personhood" at fertilization). In short, I was required to spend a good deal of extra time tracking down each and every scientific point, and correcting it through research and myriads of conversations and meetings with other scientists at NIH and elsewhere. It was important to me to straighten the science out, as these scientific observations would be the *starting point* of my philosophical deliberations.

On the other hand, I am one of those who believes that true and accurate science, philosophy, and the Scriptures would complement rather than contradict each other. As Romans 1:20 relates, "He is known by the things that are." So in my own way, as both a scientist and a realistic philosopher, I have taken this as a sort of private covenant. I resolved that once I straightened out the science, I would just see where it would lead me—and it led me to a quite different and, frankly, politically incorrect, position!

The question of when "personhood" begins is central to all of the issues in ethics and bioethics. In the context of philosophy, how one defines a human being or a human person determines what ethical choices one should make. In the context of current bioethics, it not only determines our choices about abortion, but also many other bioethical issues which are *interrelated* with abortion—especially those issues at the beginning and the end of life, such as embryo and fetal research, gene screening and therapy, and *in vitro* fertilization, or the definition of brain death, the withdrawal of food and water for a patient, allocation of scarce medical resources, and euthanasia. Virtually each person today will be dramatically and personally touched by how we, as Christians or as society at large, define a human being. Public policy is already based on *someone's* definition of a human being! The question to ask is: Is their definition correct or defensible?

This discussion will necessarily become a little technical. But I ask you to at least consider seriously the following information, for these days the contemporary social and political debates on the bioethical issues are won or lost on just these fine, seemingly esoteric scientific or philosophical points. Neither the rest of the academic community nor we as Christians can afford to remain aloof from these technical issues anymore. The good news is that the position of those Christians who believe in the inalienable dignity and personhood of the pre-born child—at all of his or her growing stages—is indeed based on quite solid scientific and philosophical grounds!

Too often we hear the claim of the relativist: "We just don't or can't know what a human being or a human person really is," or, "There just is no consensus or agreement on what the definition of a human being or a human person is, so why should one person's or one group's definition be preferred over any other? The definition of a human being or of a human person cannot be objectively determined, and so must remain a relative one."

I argue here against this relativistic claim. We can and do have an objective and empirically based definition of a human being or human person. Other than conceptually, or mentally, one cannot really split a human being from a human person. The terms are co-extensive. "Personhood" begins when the human being begins. If ever there was an example of a time when solid reasoning and scientific facts can inform the faith we already have, this is surely one.

First, I will briefly note some of the most important kinds of arguments for "delayed personhood." For example, many claim that the early human zygote, embryo, or fetus is not really a human being, but sort of like tissues or organs of the mother. Many are arguing that even if it is a human being, it is not yet a human person (and therefore deserving of the same moral and legal protections as all other human persons). Both of these kinds of arguments are blatantly incorrect and, as I will demonstrate, grounded in textbook-wrong scientific facts, as well as in passé philosophical "facts" and theories which, in philosophical jargon, contain a massive mind/body split and are empirically refuted. This mind/body split renders them theoretically and practically indefensible, as there can then be *no interaction* of any sort possible or explainable between the mind and the body.

Second, in order to draw you into the issue as quickly as possible, I want to pose a few questions to clarify exactly what is at stake when we define a human being or a human person in one way or another. To paraphrase an old philosopher: "A small error in the beginning leads to a multitude of errors in the end." In other words, if our definition of a human being or a human person is incorrect even in part, then the consequences of this incorrect definition are profound.

So I pose the question, how would you yourself define a human person? Is a rock, a tomato, or a frog a human being? Those who are old and senile in a nursing home? How about Alzheimers, Parkinsonian, stroke, comatose, or "PVS" patients? Drunks and alchoholics, drug addicts, the homeless, the poor? Prisoners, the emotionally ill and depressed, mothers-in-law, teenagers, the physically handicapped, the mentally infirm? Children under seven years of age, a newborn baby, the fetus before the mother has given birth (or, at six months, eight weeks, thirty-five days, fourteen days, six days, two days, fertilization, or the egg or the sperm)? These latter examples actually constitute some of the different biological markers at which various writers claim that there is present a human person. Obviously, there is some disagreement about exactly when we have, definitionally, a human person present. And that period of time between fertilization and about eight weeks is the grayest area, i.e., the seemingly most difficult and most controversial stage. It is particularly this period of time on which I will focus most of this discussion.

My approach to refute "delayed personhood" will be the following. First, I will lay out in very general terms the kinds of arguments offered for the so-called "biological marker events of personhood." Second, because the science and philosophy are so intertwined, I must address briefly the correct science that we do know, and that philosophical "ball park" which does realistically match that correct biology, and grounds of the argument for "immediate personhood." Third, I will point out in more detail some of the major specific arguments for "delayed personhood" and indicate their use of incorrect science and philosophy.

The Kinds of Arguments on "Personhood"

First let me brush in broad strokes the kinds of arguments for "personhood," or when, during embryological development we have a human being or a human person. There are three general categories of arguments:

A. *Fertilization.* "Personhood" begins when the human being begins, at *fertilization.* There is no distinction between a human being and a human person—they cannot be split. At some definite point in time during the process of fertilization, *substantial* change has taken place, and a new, unique, living, individual human being who is a human person is present. Embryological development, on the other hand, is not substantial change, but only *accidental* change, or continuous development in size, shape, and specialization.

B. *Physiological capacities (or preconditions) for "rational attributes" or sentience.* This argument is concerned with the actual physiological "capacity" required to be present if there is to be a human "person." "Capacity" is meant here in a rather passive sense; that is, the focus is on whatever nature is required as a *precondition* for there being a human person present. This argument (like the third one) breaks down into two types of "capacities." One is the capacity to exercise so-called *"rational attributes"* (e.g., loving, hating, willing, reasoning, interacting with the environment around one, consciousness or self-consciousness, etc.). This is a type of "rationalistic" philosophical criteria. The other is the capacity to be *sentient,* or to feel pain or pleasure. This is a type of an "empiricist" or materialistic criterion. Both criteria are based on the requirement that there is somehow a split between a human being and a human person.

C. *Exercising of the capacities for "rational attributes" or sentience.* This argument is concerned with the *actual exercising* of these capacities. Thus, some will argue that there is no person present until those "rational attributes" are actually actively operating. Others will argue there is no person present until full brain integration and full sentience is actually actively operating. What I want to stress up front is that any of the arguments from both the second and third group are biologically impossible and refutable, and that any of the arguments from the third group lead necessarily to the moral acceptance of the infanticide of perfectly normal healthy infants and children, whether one realizes this at first or not.

Interestingly enough, these three general categories of arguments actually tend to very roughly parallel a stretch of the history of philosophy: an Aristotelean, a Cartesian, and a rationalist or an empiricist school of thought. This leads to the next section, i.e., the connection between the science and the philosophy.

The Connection Between Science and Philosophy

First, although a question about "natures" seems to be fundamentally a philosophical one, any philosophical reflections, analyses or accounts about the nature of a human being or person must begin with the empirically observable biological facts.[2] Otherwise our philosophical concepts actually bear little or no relation or resemblance to the real world which we are trying to understand and explain by those concepts. Instead, we are left with multiple half-truths or fantasies—or wishful thinking! A realistic or objectively based definition of a human being—one that is not relativistic—must start with these empirical facts.

Operationally, what is the connection between a thing's nature and the biological facts? Put briefly, the answer is that we can know *what* a thing is, i.e., its *nature,* by observing its *actions* or *functions*—how it behaves, what it does. We know that a thing acts according to the *kind* of thing it is, i.e., its nature. In first-year chemistry, microbiology, or genetics, students are given "unknowns" which they must identify by means of the kinds of actions or reactions exhibited by these "unknowns." Thus sodium burns orange, and cobalt burns blue/green. Beta-hemolytic streptococcus can only be grown on specific culture medium containing blood, but not on other mediums. And a particular member of a plant or animal species is identified microscopically by the number of chromosomes present in a single cell. Indeed, this is the obvious principle behind any basic or experimental research. The research biologist first observes the actions, reactions, *functions* of a biological entity and reasons from these specific *kinds* of actions back to the specific kind of *nature* it possesses. It is this nature which directs and causes such characteristic actions. As biology texts themselves discuss it: Function follows form.[3]

Further, a thing is not only characterized by its nature, which determines the specific kinds of actions it can do, but that same nature limits the kinds of actions it can do. That is, there are certain actions which a thing cannot do because it does not have the specific kind of nature it would need to do it. For example, birds have wings and so can fly; but stones, dogs, or human beings can't fly. Corn stalks produce ears of corn and corn proteins and corn enzymes; but acorns, tomato plants or asteroids do not and cannot produce corn or corn proteins. Frog embryos direct the formation of frog tissues and organs, but they cannot direct the formation of human tissues and organs.

Application to Scientific Facts of Human Fertilization

Apply these considerations to the point at hand. To determine what a human being or person is is really not all so difficult as is often claimed. There are voluminous biological facts which we do know already about the human body and its embryological development. Clearly, by observing and studying these known biological facts—how the human being begins his or her biological existence as a specifically *human* zygote, and the kinds of specifically *human functions* and *human actions* that take place during embryological development—we can then determine to a very sophisticated extent the nature of a human being or a human embryo, or what it is. So I will turn now to a brief consideration of the biological facts about which most, if not all, of us are already aware.

Before fertilization there exist a human sperm (containing "23" chromosomes) and a human ovum or egg (also containing "23" chromosomes—the same number, but different kinds of chromosomes).[4] Neither the sperm nor the egg can, by itself, become a human being, even if implanted in the womb of the mother. They are only gametes, not human embryos or human beings. In contrast, the single-cell human zygote formed after fertilization, or syngamy, contains "46" chromosomes (the number of chromosomes which is specific for members of the human species), and these 46 chromosomes are mixed differently from the "46" chromosomes as found in the mother or in the father—that is, they are unique for that human individual. This is why an embryo or fetus is not just a tissue or organ of the mother! Thus, with fertilization *substantial* change has taken place, i.e., a change in *natures,* as observable by the different kinds of functions and actions which now take place. If allowed to "do his or her own thing," so to speak, this human zygote (who is already a he or a she!) will biologically develop *itself* continuously without any biological gaps throughout the embryonic, fetal, neonatal, childhood, and adulthood stages until the death of the organism.

I want to reiterate that a human gamete is not a human being or a human person. The number of chromosomes is only "23"; it only acts or functions biologically as an egg or as a sperm; e.g., it only makes egg or sperm enzymes and proteins, etc., not specifically human enzymes and proteins; and by itself it does not have the actual capacity or potency yet to develop into a human embryo, fetus, child, or adult. (And in that sense *gametes* are only possible human beings, i.e., nonexistent human beings). Only after the sperm and the egg chromosomes combine properly and completely do we have an existing human being.

After fertilization there is not substantial change, but only *accidental* change.[5] That is, during embryogenesis the nature of the human being does not change, only its accidents change (e.g., size, shape, color, etc.). Once it is a human being, it stays a human being, and acts and functions biologically as a human being from the start. The human zygote itself produces specifically human enzymes and proteins; he or she forms specifically human tissues and organ systems, and develops itself humanly and continuously from the stage of a human single-cell zygote to the stage of a human adult.[6] This is observed empirically.[7] A human zygote does not produce cabbage or carrot enzymes or proteins, and does not develop into a rock, an ear of corn, nor into a cat, a horse, a chicken, or a giraffe. He or she develops continuously throughout embryological development in a specifically and characteristically human way.

In short, the biological facts demonstrate that at least by syngamy we have a truly *human* nature. It is not that he or she will *become* a human being, that he or she is a *possible* or a *potential* human being. He or she already *is* a human being. We know that empirically. And this nature or capacity to act in a certain characteristic way is called, philosophically, a nature or a *potency*.[8] This is the classical term which has been so seriously misused in the recent "personhood" debates. A human zygote or embryo is not a possible human being;[9] nor is he or she a potential human being;[10] he or she *is* a human being with a potency (or potential) to further develop (or grow) itself.

Now, this is irrefutable empirical evidence that at least by syngamy there is a human being; but is there also a human person— or not? It is in this shifting from the paradigm of a human being to that of a human person where the philosophy comes into play again. Is a human being also a human person, or are they different things? Which philosophy is adequate to cope with this biological data?

With even a cursory rummaging through the history of philosophy, there is one major "realistic" philosophical "ball park" which would deny any real essential distinction between a human being and a human person—they cannot be split or separated from each other, except perhaps only *conceptually*. This philosophy was part of a 2,500-year-old tradition which was the bath water, so to speak, that was "thrown out with the baby"! It is the philosophical ball park, for example, of Aristotle-the-biologist.[11]

For Aristotle, as well as for others, his major metaphysical and anthropological treatises argue consistently for a human substance with no mind/body split (although there is evidence of a serious Platonic streak in his *De Anima*—that atypical and historically problematic treatise of Aristotle's—followed unblushingly by some, and so often quoted by contemporary scholars, as well as historians who researched for *Roe v. Wade*). In an Aristotelean "ball park," matter cannot exist apart from the form—at least not in this world. The human being is defined as one composite substance—the vegetative, sensitive, and rational powers of the "soul" together with the human "body."[12] The whole "soul," he wrote, is homogenous, and in each part of the body as one whole composite:

> In each of the bodily parts there are present *all* the parts of the soul, and the souls so present are homogenous with one another and with the whole; this means

33

that the several parts of the soul are *indisseverable* from one another.[13] (emphasis added)

This means that the "soul" is not a separately existing substance in itself, nor is it found in any one particular organ, e.g., the heart or the brain. And Aristotle addresses the very possibility of a "being-on-the-way," or an "intermediate human being," railing against the anthropological consequences of Plato's or Pythagoras' mind/body split when he very sarcastically retorts: "Yet how are we to believe in such things?"[14] Although Aristotle-proper did not actually use the term "person," he clearly would have to concur that a human being is always a human person, for neither form nor matter can exist on their own in this life as two different things or independent substances. Rather, matter and form (or the soul and the body) are two different aspects of *one* thing.

Another philosopher puts an even finer gloss on Aristotle's anthropology. To paraphrase him: "The name of *'person'* [and he uses that term] does not belong to the rational part of the soul alone, nor to the whole soul alone, but to the entire human substance (or, subsistens)."[15] This means that the whole soul, whole body, and its act of existing constitutes *one* personal substance entire, with no separate and troublesome independent "parts" which are claimed to be true and independent substances themselves.

In this philosophical "ball park," then, a human being is a human person; the terms are co-extensive. And the later characteristics which we will look at in these debates, such as "rational attributes," autonomous willing or sentience, are really only consequential and secondary or accidental *actions* which follow upon certain sensitive or rational *powers* which themselves follow upon the essential *nature* of the human being itself.[16] That nature is defined as the single, whole, formal, material and existential human substance. The nature of a human being, then, is not defined in terms of only one aspect of the soul (e.g., the "rational" aspect), or in terms of any one activity of the soul, but in terms of the *whole complex human being*. As it is put:

. . . the soul must be in the whole body [and therefore not just in the brain], and in each part thereof . . . for to the nature of the species belongs what the definition signifies; and in natural things, the *definition* does not signify the form only, but the form *and* the matter . . . so it belongs to the notion of man to be composed of soul, flesh and bones.[17] (emphasis added)

What significance does this have for the arguments for "delayed personhood"? If it is claimed that the "rational" soul—which "organizes and directs embryological development"—is not infused until sometime up to about the third month,[18] then what explains the specifically *human* organization of the human embryo and human fetus up to that point? Hasn't the work of this supposed "delayed rational soul" already been done, as empirically verified? If so, then this biological evidence of specifically human *organization* which we do empirically observe must be accounted for by the presence of the human ("rational") soul right from the beginning. We also empirically observe specifically *human* functions and activities from the beginning—e.g., the production of specifically human proteins, enzymes, etc. If so, then this biological evidence of specifically human *functions and activities* which we do empirically observe must be accounted for by the presence of the human ("rational") soul right from the beginning.

Again, this human "rational" soul must *include* virtually the vegetative and sensitive powers,[19] for there is no such thing, at least in this earthly life, as a part of a "rational soul" alone, or even a whole soul alone as a complete human being. The whole human complex (body and soul) must be present together at once. At least I have never seen a human being on this planet who did not have a body! And apart from the biological and conceptual absurdity of an "intermediate human being," if there were only a "human vegetative" soul present at first, how do we explain the production of specifically human enzymes and proteins (instead of carrot or corn enzymes) from the very start? If there were only a "human vegetative and sensitive" soul present, how do we explain the production of specifically human tissue and organs instead of giraffe or gorilla organs and systems? If the human soul cannot be split (and must contain all three powers at once), and if specifically human enzymes, proteins, tissues, organs and structures are empirically observed—which they are—then the human *rational* soul must be present at the very beginning along *with* the human vegetative and sensitive "powers" of the human soul. And these powers must exist as a composite with the human body which it is organizing and whose functions and activities it is directing. Thus, at least by syngamy the "matter" is already appropriately organized as human; we empirically observe it as human and as developing humanly.[20]

Incorrect Scientific Arguments for Delayed Personhood

So far the scientific facts and the philosophical concepts match. At this point I want to take a closer look at the biological facts after fertilization, i.e., those of human embryological development. Along the way I will point out several other different biological "marker events" of personhood which have been argued by others. All of these writers will make a *distinction* between a human being and a human person, supposedly based on these biological marker events. The use of certain biological data which they will use to support their arguments will also be addressed.

Capacity for "Rational Attributes" or Sentience

As noted above, the newly formed single-cell human zygote consists of "46" chromosomes and non-nuclear DNA in which are coded the specific directions for virtually *all* of the processes of embryological development. The content of this initial pool of genetic information *never changes* throughout embryological development.

(1) However, it has been argued[21] [22] that not all of the "information" needed is present in this single original cell, that some of the information comes from "positional molecules" in later stages of development, and some even comes from molecules originating from the mother. They conclude that the original human zygote does *not* contain all of the information needed to be a self-directing human individual, and therefore it is neither a human being nor a human person.

This biological data is inaccurate. First, "molecular information" or "positional information" is simply not the same as genetic information—what the fertilization argument is talking about. Also, molecular or positional information is itself coded in the original single-cell human zygote. As the well-known embryologist Moore discusses at great length, the genetic information in the original human zygote itself determines what molecules will be formed, which in turn determine what proteins and enzymes will be formed, which in turn determine which tissues and organs will be formed. In genetics this is called the "cascading effect."[23] That is, the information in the original single-cell human zygote "cascades" throughout embryological development, each previous direction causing the specific formation of each succeeding direction. Thus, all "positional" or "molecular" information or direction is already determined itself by the information which preceded it, and ultimately by the original information in the single-cell human zygote.

Second, although the information in the human zygote may direct the absorption of molecules from the mother, that hardly means that the maternal molecules or the mother herself determines the very nature of the growing embryo or fetus which she is nurturing.[24] The nature of the embryo or fetus, we know, is determinable and set by the formal biological genetic make-up of the zygote from which he or she continuously develops, and the directing of this absorption or use of maternal molecules is done by the genetic information within the embryo or fetus, not by the mother. Those are simply the correct biological facts. As Jerome Lejeune, the internationally renowned human geneticist has testified:

> . . . each of us has a unique beginning, the moment of conception. . . . As soon as the twenty-three chromosomes carried by the sperm encounter the twenty-three chromosomes carried by the ovum, the *whole information* necessary and sufficient to spell out all the characteristics of the new being is gathered. . . .[25] (emphasis added)

Finally, it is argued that hydatiform moles and teratomas (which are not human beings) can be produced by the human zygote, and therefore the human zygote is not a human being. But hydatiform moles and teratomas arise from chromosomally abnormal entities to begin with, not from normal human embryos.[26]

(2) Next, others argue for the presence of the "rational human nature" at the two-cell stage, with the completion of the first division and the *completion of the genetic input*. The two-cell stage already is, like the adult, a moment in the execution of the program "man"; and it is already the *same* living being as the human adult arising from it.[27] However, we already know that the genetic input is complete at the *zygote* stage, and that the zygote in fact is the source of the genetic input of the two-cell stage. We also know that the zygote, too, is the same living being as both the two-cell stage and the adult stage. Thus their argument actually argues for the *zygote* rather than for his two-cell stage!

(3) Next, it is argued that this original single cell divides neatly first into two cells, then into four cells, then into eight cells, etc.[28] This biological data, too, is inaccurate, and has consequences in understanding the argument about "totipotency." As known and published in embryological textbooks for over sixty years,[29] the original single cell divides into two cells, and then only one of those cells divides, giving three cells. After a time the other cell divides, making it four cells, and then eight cells, etc.

Part of what happens at this three-cell stage is that one can observe empirically the process of methylation. This observation is important philosophically. Many argue that these very early cells, including the original single-cell zygote up to the eight-cell stage, are "totipotent." They explain totipotent cells as the most vaguely directed and least differentiated cells in all of embryological development. Each cell is not yet determined enough to be classified as an individual human being or a part of an individual human being. These cells, they say, have not yet "made up their minds" what they want to be. They can become any number of things. These cells are not differentiated or specialized enough yet.

This portrayal of totipotency, differentiation, and specialization is conceptually confusing, incorrect, scientifically simplistic, and backwards. For example, not all totipotent cells have the *same* "potential." And as Lejeune notes, totipotent cells are the *most* determined and most specialized cells in all of development *because* they are the least differentiated. Progressively the developing cells lose, in fact, the ability to *use* this information. In embryological development no information is lost, only the ability to use the information is lost.[30] To take an extreme example, a kidney cell contains virtually all of the information that was in the original single human zygote cell. The kidney cell has not lost any of this information—only the ability to use this information. This ability to use or not use the information that is present results in differentiation. And differentiation is partially determined by the process of methylation (which itself is coded in the original single-cell zygote). Through methylation and other processes during embryogenesis, genes are turned on or turned off. When the cell wants to control the use of cellular information, it methylates a molecule to silence that gene, to block or stop its use at a certain point in development. It is this process of methylation which we can empirically observe the human embryo directing at the three-cell stage.

Thus to be so differentiated as a kidney cell is actually a negative in such arguments. The kidney cell cannot direct anything but a small miniscule part of the development of the human embryo or fetus, whereas the original totipotent human zygote contains and can use all of the information only partially used by the later cells. Thus there is nothing vague, undirected or undecided about being totipotent.[31] Totipotent cells are supposed to be undifferentiated because they are so "all-specialized." Totipotency is supposed to happen—it is a normal part of human embryogenesis, and is indeed encoded in the original genetic information of the human zygote, as is differentiation. Differentiation, then, really represents the *restricted* ability to make any "decisions," a characteristic which totipotent cells do not want.

(4) But to continue, the cells will proceed to divide until about five or six days, when two cell layers are formed—the trophoblast or outer cell layer, and the blastocyst or inner cell layer. Some claim that there can be no true human individual present at this time; we have only a genetic individual, not a *developmental* individual. Only a "developmental individual" can be a person.[32] These early cells are only "collections" of undifferentiated cells, and they name them, or designate them collectively, as only comprising a "pre-embryo" (a term, by the way, which is not used by embryologists—only by philosophers, theologians and bioethicists).

Scientific facts which they give to support these claims are the following. Only the cells from the inner layer, the blastocyst, eventually become the adult human being. The cells from the trophoblast layer are *all discarded after birth* as the sac and the umbilical cord, etc. Thus, developmentally, the implication is that we are not dealing only with those important cells which will become the adult human being, i.e., the blastocyst, but rather a mixture of "essential" and "nonessential" cells, i.e., a *pre*-embryo. A pre-embryo is not even a human being yet, much less a human person.[33]

But, again, these scientific "facts" are inaccurate, and necessarily lead to incorrect philosophical concepts. It simply is not true that all of the cells from the trophoblast layer are discarded after birth. As can be found in virtually all embryology texts, many of the cells from this trophoblast layer become an integral and essential part of the constitution of the fetus, newborn, and adult human being. For example, the cells from the trophoblast layer known as the yolk sac cells become part of the adult gut. And cells known as the allantois cells become part of the adult ligaments, blood cells and urinary bladder.[34]

Thus their "scientific" facts are inaccurate—and so, therefore, are their philosophical conclusions about "pre-embryos" and "developmental individuals" which are grounded on those inaccurate scientific facts.

But the same writers continue. It is impossible for a human person to be present until at least the fourteen-day marker event, at which point the primitive streak forms in the embryo. The philosophical significance of this marker is that until the formation of the primitive streak it is possible for *twinning* to take place. The totipotent cells "do not yet know whether to be one or two individuals." After fourteen days, they claim, twinning is *not possible,* and thus the organism is finally, "developmentally" one individual.[35]

But, again, this science is inaccurate. As Karen Dawson[36] and others point out in these debates—and as is found in every human genetics textbook—it *is* possible for monozygotic twinning to take place after fourteen days and the formation of the primitive streak. For example, fetus-in-fetu twins can be formed up to two and three months after fertilization, and Siamese twins even later. There is nothing magical, it turns out, about this fourteen-day stage as far as the concept of individuality and personhood is concerned. If a two-cell, eight-cell, implantation stage, fourteen-day primitive streak stage embryo or four-month fetus splits into twins, that simply means that the original entity was already one individual, and now there are simply two individuals. The fact of twinning says nothing about the individuality of the first individual. Indeed, the history of all living organisms is of one individual giving rise to another individual, but one would certainly not then conclude that there were therefore no individuals ever present, or that the former individual was hopelessly "undecided."

(5) Many others[37] also argue for the fourteen-day stage, *based primarily on the same science as above.* Although they would agree that there is an individual present at fertilization, it is only a biological individual. Rational ensoulment cannot take place until after fourteen days, at which point there is an *ontological* individual, i.e., when *differentiation is completed* and thus a distinct individuality.[38] But aside from the problems with the above inaccurate science on which they base their own claims, complete differentiation does not actually take place until well *after birth.* As the embryologist Moore explains:

> Human development is a continuous process that begins when an ovum from a female is fertilized by a sperm from a male. Growth and differentiation transform the zygote, a single cell formed by the union of the ovum and the sperm, into a multicellular adult human being. Most developmental changes occur during the embryonic and the fetal periods, but important [developmental] changes also occur during the other periods of development: childhood, adolescence, and adulthood. . . . Although it is customary to divide development into prenatal and postnatal periods, it is important to realize that birth is merely a dramatic event during development resulting in a distinct change in environment.

> Development does not stop at birth: important develop-
> mental changes, in addition to growth, occur after birth.
> . . . Most developmental changes are completed by *the
> age of 25*.[39]

Thus differentiation and development are not really completed until *well* after birth. Certainly a *fourteen-day embryo* is definitely *not* completely differentiated.

(6) Still other writers argue for fourteen days because the formation of the primitive streak signals the beginning of sentience (or the ability to feel pain). However, it will become clear below that true sentience is also not complete until well after birth.

(7) Another argument is that "personhood" does not begin until the dawning of or the maturation of the physical substrate of human consciousness, self-consciousness, or sentience, i.e., the formation of the nervous system and/or the brain (about eight weeks or several time-markers after that). But the fact is that complete physiological brain integration is not complete until many *months or years after birth,*[40] just as the complete exercising of "rational attributes" is not possible until years after birth.[41]

Yet there is already a movement by some in legal jurisprudence to formalize the legal concept of "brain birth" to denote that point in time biologically when there is present a "person," as a *parallel* to the already legal criteria of brain death.[42] Criticisms of these claims come, for example, from Gareth Jones, a neurologist, who rejects the arguments that we can determine the biological point of either "rational attributes" or sentience. As he states, the parallelism between brain death and brain birth is invalid. Brain death is the gradual or rapid cessation of the functions of a brain. Brain birth is the very gradual acquisition of the functions of a developing neural system. This developing neural system is *not* a brain. He questions, in fact, the entire assumption and retorts that there are *no* physiological neurological reasons for concluding that an incapacity for consciousness becomes a capacity for consciousness once this point is passed! Jones continues that the alleged symmetry is not as strong as is sometimes assumed, and that it has yet to be provided with a firm biological base![43]

Thus, in all of these arguments the science used is inaccurate, and therefore their conclusions about "delayed personhood" are invalid. It must also be stressed that the functional physiological precondition for either "rational attributes" or sentience is the one-cell human zygote itself.

Exercising Capacity for "Rational Attributes"

Examples of the third category of arguments include claims that personhood requires the actual *exercising* of the capacity for "rational attributes" or for sentience.

(1) When the focus is "rational attributes," a "person" is defined necessarily as a young child or adult, and the *infanticide* of normal, healthy infants is openly acknowledged and promoted. This can be found in the writings of Hare, Engelhardt, and Tooley.[44]

(2) Many who argue for sentience often define some animals as "persons" and some human beings as "nonpersons." Here they have pushed such above rationalistic definitions to their logical limits. For example, Peter Singer (yes, the animal rights person) argues in the literature for sentience, and therefore for the infanticide of even a normal, healthy infant.[45] If, he argues, a normal newborn baby cannot act rationally (as described above), then it is not a subject but only an object, and we can therefore use it in destructive experimental research if we rational agents so choose. In Singer's own words:

> Now it must be admitted that these arguments apply to the newborn baby as much as to the fetus. A week-old baby is not a rational and self-conscious being, and there are many nonhuman animals whose rationality, self-consciousness, awareness, capacity to feel pain (sentience), and so on, exceed that of a human baby a week, a month, or even a year old. If the fetus does not have the same claim to life as a person, [then] it appears that the *newborn baby is of less value than the life of a pig, a dog, or a chimpanzee.*[46] (emphasis added)

And finally, an example of the arguments for sentience or whole brain integration in this third category of arguments leads necessarily to the same conclusion (i.e., infanticide), because full sentience or full brain integration does not take place until well *after birth*.

Discussion of Personhood

I could continue, biologically, down dozens of "marker events" where it is argued at different points during biological development that until that point there is only a human being and only after that point there is a human person. But virtually every single marker event claimed is also using extremely problematic scientific "data" to back up their *philosophical* claims of personhood. It would seem that there is more of a problem here than simply the use of problematic science. Perhaps there is also involved, whether consciously or not, the imposition on that science of certain characteristically problematic philosophical presuppositions. What I see is the use of specific metaphysical presuppositions which result in a classic mind/body split. Thus a rough consideration of just how other philosophical schools of thought have defined a "human being" or a "human person" might be helpful. Especially in light of the obvious biological continuity present throughout the entire course of embryological development, as well as the specifically human development which we know empirically takes place, how adequately do the other philosophical definitions of a human person reflect or match the correct biological facts as we empirically know them?

I will focus on the definition that is most generally agreed upon these days, i.e., one that is basically "derived" from Descartes[47] or Locke.[48] Generally, a human "person" is someone who is *actually acting* at the time in a rational manner. That is, he or she is self-conscious, self-aware, competent, autonomous, logical, mature, conversant, and interacts with the environment and other rational beings around him or her. In short, if one is *acting rationally,* one is a person. If this is true, then 99 percent of the possible examples of human persons I gave you at the beginning of this chapter are by definition *not persons,* and therefore not deserving of moral or legal protections!

Would you agree that the killing of normal, healthy, human newborns is morally justifiable? If not, then we have to question, at least, such very rationalistic definitions of a human person, and the metaphysical and epistemological foundations on which they are grounded. If one agrees with the rationalistic premise that a "human person" is defined only in terms of "active reason," then you must agree with Singer's and others' arguments for infanticide. Furthermore, any Cartesian or rationalist definition of a human being as composed of two independently existing substances collapses, since there is absolutely *no interaction possible* between the physical substrate (e.g., the brain) and the immaterial Mind or Reason.

On the other hand, sometimes a human "person" is defined only in terms of the *whole soul,* i.e., the vegetative, sensitive, and rational "souls" all together. Once this soul unites with a body, we then have a human person. It doesn't matter, they say, whether this person is presently acting rationally. What is important is that the rational *capacity* is present. But if we think about it, we run into similar problems as mentioned earlier. If there are no vegetative, sensitive, or rational directions injected until about three months, how did a specifically human biochemical, tissue, organ system get built before three months?

Or perhaps we should restrict ourselves to a purely *material* or physical definition of a human "person." The human person is simply a complex system of molecules, tissues, and organs. But this definition has continuously failed in explaining our experience of thoughts, ideas, and concepts, and especially of intentionality, willing, or choosing. It is argued that a "person" is simply a more advanced sophisticated *phase* of a complex material human being. But aren't we really talking then about a secondary or *accidental* quality? Surely the definition of the *nature* of a human person should not be put in terms of only a secondary or accidental phase, however sophisticated it may be. And again, if you are arguing from the materialist premise that a human "person" is defined only in terms of sentience, or the physical integration or functioning of the brain, then you too will have to argue for infanticide, because as pointed out, full physical integration and sentience is not completed until several years after birth.

Conclusions

Given the scientific and philosophical problems inherent in the positions which argue for the various biological marker events of "personhood," can we really accept their conclusions? Are they reconcilable with the correct biological facts? Can you really have a human person without simultaneously having a human being? And vice versa, can you really have a human being without also simultaneously having a human person?

I would argue no—you really can't split them (except conceptually), as rationalistic or empiricist philosophers are wont to do. And delayed hominization simply does not match up with the correct empirical facts. The definition of a human "being" or a human "person" does not have to be relative, as long as the correct science is employed, and our philosophical definitions actually match that reality. In sum, if given the straight facts, we know that every human being is a human person from fertilization on. But, of course, faith-filled Christians already know that!

Endnotes

[1]Much of this material is drawn from my doctoral dissertation [Dianne Nutwell Irving, Ph.D., *Philosophical and Scientific*

Analysis of the Nature of the Early Human Embryo (Georgetown University, 1991)]; "Scientific and philosophical expertise: An evaluation of the arguments on 'personhood,'" *Linacre Quarterly* 60(1) (Feb. 1993), 18-46; "The impact of scientific misinformation on other fields: Philosophy, theology, biomedical ethics, public policy," *Accountability in Research* 2(4) (Feb. 1993), 243-272.

[2]Aristotle, *Categories,* in Sir David Ross, *Aristotle* (New York: Random House, 1985), 20-21; also, Aristotle, *Analytica Posteriora* 2.19, 100a 3-9, in Richard McKeon (ed.), *The Basic Works of Aristotle* (New York: Random House, 1941); for Aquinas's similar position, see: *The Division and Method of the Sciences,* Q6, a.1, reply to 1st Q, 65-66; ibid., Q6, reply to 3rd Q, 71-72; ibid., Q6, a.2, 176-178; ibid., Q6, a.4, 90; ibid., Q5, a.3, 35 (also quoted there in note 21: *In I Post. Anal.* lect. 1-3, and in *De Veritate* 1.1); see also George Klubertanz, *Introduction to the Philosophy of Being* (New York: Appleton-Century-Crofts, 1963), 293-298.

[3]Benjamin Lewin (ed.), *Genes III* (New York: John Wiley and Sons, 1987), 11-13, 17-19, 30, 32, 33, 35, 37, 79, 91, 93-94; also Alan E.H. Emery, *Elements of Medical Genetics* (New York: Churchill Livingstone, 1983), 25, 34, 65, 101-103.

[4]Keith L. Moore, *The Developing Human,* 3rd ed. (Philadelphia: W.B. Saunders Company, 1982), 14ff; also Benjamin Lewin, *Genes III* (New York: John Wiley and Sons, 1987), 24ff.

[5]Aristotle, "Physica," (McKeon, 1941): 1.7.191a, 15-18, 232-233; also, 2.3.194b, 23-25, 240-241; See also Henry B. Veatch, *Aristotle: A Contemporary Approach* (Indiana: Indiana University Press, 1974), chaps. 2, 3; for Thomas Aquinas, see George Klubertanz, *The Philosophy of Human Nature* (New York: Appleton-Century-Crofts, 1953), 124ff; also G. Klubertanz, *Introduction to the Philosophy of Being* (New York: Appleton-Century-Crofts, 1963), 98-100, 116 (and Thomas Aquinas, *Commentary on Aristotle's Metaphysics,* Bk. VIII, lect. 1, Cathala (ed.), Nos. 1688-1689, as quoted 118).

[6]See Moore (1982) and Lewin (1987), note 4.

[7]Irving, *Philosophical and Scientific Analysis...*(1991), see notes 78-80. There is a rapidly increasing volume of this kind of work, e.g., Kollias, G.; Hurst, J.; deBoer, E.; and Grosveld, F. "The human beta-globulin gene contains a downstream developmental specific enhancer," *Nucleic Acids Research* 15(14) (July 1987), 5739-47; R.K. Humphries, et al, "Transfer of human and murine globin-gene sequences into transgenic mice," *American Journal of Human Genetics* 37(2) (1985), 295-310; A. Schnieke et al. "Introduction of the human pro alpha 1 (I) collagen gene into pro

alpha 1 (I) - deficient Mov-13 mouse cells leads to formation of functional mouse-human hybrid type I collagen," *Proceedings of the National Academy of Science - USA* 84(3) (Feb. 1987), 764-768.

[8]See note 5 *supra.*

[9]*pace* R.M. Hare, "When does potentially count? A comment on Lockwood," *Bioethics* 2(3), 1988.

[10]*pace* Michael Lockwood, "Warnock versus Powell (and Harradine): When does potentiality count?" *Bioethics* 2(3), 1988.

[11]For brevity I will designate Aristotle's theory of substance as a *composite,* which is the predominant one in his *Categories, Physics*, the first half of the *Metaphysics*, and even in many parts of his *De Anima*, as "Aristotle-proper." Aristotle's theory of substance as *form alone,* or as only the *"rational"* part of the form, and the succession of souls as found predominantly in the second half of his *Metaphysics* and in parts of the *De Anima*, contradicts the former theory. There is also some degree of contradiction in Thomas, insofar as he sometimes "unblushingly" follows Aristotle's theory of separate form (see, for example, the differences between the definition of a human being and that of a human soul in the *De Ente et Essentia* in Chapter Two and Chapter Four).

[12]Aristotle, *De Anima* 1.5.411b, 14-18, (McKeon, 1941), 554.

[13]Aristotle, *De Anima*, 1.5.411b, 24-28, (McKeon, 1941), 554.

[14]Aristotle, *Metaphysics*, 3.2.997b18-998a10, (McKeon, 1941), 721; see also 11.1.1059a34-1059b14. 850-851; for Aquinas, see ST, Ia.q.45, a.4, ad.2, 235.

[15]Thomas Aquinas, ST, Ia.q29, a.1, ans., ad.2,3,5, 156; ibid, a.2, ans., 157; also ST, IIIa.q19, a.1, ad.4.2127; see also, Kevin Doran, "Person: a key concept for ethics," *Linacre Quarterly* 56(4), 1989, 39.

[16]Thomas Aquinas, ST, IIIa. q19, a.1, ad.4.2127; see also Kevin Doran (1989), 39.

[17]Thomas Aquinas, ST, Ia.q75, a.4, ans., 366.

[18]For example, Suarez, McCormick, Ford and Bole, *infra.*

[19]Aristotle, *De Anima*, 1.5.411b, 14-18, (McKeon, 1941), 554; also, 1.5.411b, 24-28, 554; for Thomas Aquinas, see *Summa Theologica*, Fathers of the English Dominican Province (trans.) (Westminster, Maryland: Christian Classics, Vols. 1, 2, 1989): Ia.q29, a.1, ans., ad.2,3,5, 156; ibid., a.2, ans., p. 157; also, IIIa.q19, a.1. ad.4.2127; see also Kevin Doran, "Person: a key concept for ethics," *Linacre Quarterly* 56(4), 1989, 39.

[20]As Klubertanz has expressed it, the human soul, being a form, cannot be divided. The ovum and sperm unite, "thus giving rise to a single cell with the *material disposition required* for the

presence of a soul": Klubertanz, *The Philosophy of Nature*, 1953, 312.

[21]Carlos Bedate and Robert Cefalo, "The zygote: to be or not be a person," *Journal of Medicine and Philosophy* 14(6), 1989, 641-645.

[22]Thomas J. Bole, III, "Metaphysical accounts of the zygote as a person and the veto power of facts," *Journal of Medicine and Philosophy* 14, 1989: 647-653; also, "Zygotes, souls, substances, and persons," *Journal of Medicine and Philosophy* 15, 1990: 637-652.

[23]Benjamin Lewin (ed.), *Genes III* (New York: John Wiley and Sons, 1983), 681; also Alan E. H. Emery, *Elements of Medical Genetics* (New York: Churchill Livingstone, 1983), 93.

[24]H. Holtzer, J. Biekl, and B. Holtzer, "Indiction-dependent and lineage-dependent models for cell-diversification are mutually exclusive," *Progress in Clinical Biological Research* 175 (1985), 3-11; also rejected by Antoine Suarez, "Hyditiform moles and teratomas confirm the human identity of the preimplantation embryo," *Journal of Medicine and Philosophy* 15 (1990), 630. Antoine Suarez, "Hydatidiform moles and teratomas confirm the human identity of the preimplantaion embryo," *Journal of Medicine and Philosophy* 15, 1990, 630.

[25]Jerome Lejeune, testimony in *Davis v. Davis,* Circuit Court for Blount County, State of Tennessee at Maryville, Tennessee, 1989; as reprinted in Martin Palmer, *A Symphony of the Pre-Born Child: Part Two* (Hagerstown, Md.: NAAPC, 1989), 9-10.

[26]See Suarez, op. cit.

[27]Antoine Suarez, "Hydatidiform moles and teratomas confirm the human identity of the preimplantation embryo," *Journal of Medicine and Philosophy* 15 (1990): 631.

[28]See, e.g., Richard McCormick, S.J., "Who or what is the pre-embryo?" paper presented at the Andre E. Hellegers Lecture (Washington, D.C., Georgetown University: May 17, 1990); (pre-publication manuscript); see also, McCormick, "Who or what is the preembryo?" *Kennedy Institute of Ethics Journal* 1(1), 1991, 3.

[29]Lejeune, 1989, 14.

[30]Lejeune, 1989, 17, 20; also see article by Mavilio, where he explains that the modulation of the methylation pattern represents a key mechanism for regulating the expression of human globin genes during embryonic, fetal, and adult development in humans. Mavilio et al. "Molecular mechanisms of human hemoglobin switching: selective undermethylation and expression of globin genes in embryonic, fetal and adult erythroblasts," *Proceedings of*

the National Academy of Sciences USA, 80(22) (1983): 690;7-11;
see also Alan E.H. Emery, *Elements of Medical Genetics* (New
York: Churchill Livingstone, 1983), 103.

[31]See references on "cascading" in note 23, *supra*; also "transgenic mice" in note 7, *supra*.

[32]McCormick (1991), 3.

[33]3bid., 3.

[34]Keith L. Moore, *The Developing Human* (Philadelphia: W.B.
Saunders Co., 1982), 33, 62-63, 68, 111, 127; also see K. Chada et
al. "An embryonic pattern of expression of a human fetal globin
gene in transgenic mice," *Nature* 319(6055), 1986: 685-9; also G.
Migliaccio et al. "Human embryonic hemopoiesis. Kinetics of pro-
genitors and precursor underlying the yolk sac - liver transition,"
Journal of Clinical Investigation 78(1), 1986: 51-60.

[35]McCormick (1991), 4.

[36]Karen Dawson, "Segmentation and moral status," in Peter
Singer et al. *Embryo Experimentation* (New York: Cambridge
University Press, 1990), 58; see also Keith Moore (1982), 133.

[37]Norman Ford, *When Did I Begin?* (New York: Cambridge
University Press, 1988), 298.

[38]Ibid., 156.

[39]Keith L. Moore, *The Developing Human* (1982), 1.

[40]G. Gareth Jones, "Brain birth and personal identity," *Journal
of Medical Ethics* 15(4), 1989, 177.

[41]For example, see Singer and Engelhardt, *infra*.

[42]John A. Robertson, "Extracorporeal embryos and the abortion
debate," *Journal of Contemporary Health Law and Policy* 2(53),
1986, 53-70.

[43]D. Gareth Jones, "Brain birth and personal identity," *Journal
of Medical Ethics* 15(4), 1989, 178. Oddly enough Jones will himself argue for personhood at 6-7 months (p. 177).

[44]R.M. Hare, "When does potentiality count? A comment on
Lockwood", *Bioethics* 2(3) (July 1988), 214; H.T. Engelhardt, *The
Foundations of Bioethics* (New York: Oxford University Press,
1985), 111; Michael Tooley, "Abortion and infanticide," in Marshall
Cohen et al. (eds.), *The Rights and Wrongs of Abortion*, (New
Jersey: Princeton University Press, 1974), 59, 64.

[45]Peter Singer, "Taking life: abortion," in *Practical Ethics*
(London: Cambridge University Press, 1981), 123-124; see also,
Helga Kuhse and Peter Singer, "For sometimes letting—and help-
ing—die," *Law, Medicine and Health Care* 3(4), 1986: 149-153; also
Kuhse and Singer, *Should the Baby Live? The Problem of
Handicapped Infants* (Oxford: Oxford University Press, 1985), 138;

also, Peter Singer and Helga Kuhse, "The ethics of embryo research," *Law, Medicine and Health Care* 14(13-14), 1987. For one reaction, see Gavin J. Fairbairn, "Kuhse, Singer and slippery slopes," *Journal of Medical Ethics* 14 (1988), 134.

[46]Peter Singer, "Taking life: abortion" (1981), 118.

[47]Rene Descartes, *Meditations on First Philosophy*, in John Cottingham, Robert Stoothoff and Dugald Murdoch (trans.), *The Philosophical Writings of Descartes* (New York: Press Syndicate of the University of Cambridge, 1984), 2nd Meditation, 12ff.

[48]John Locke, *An Essay Concerning Human Understanding*, A.D. Woozley (ed.) (London: Fontana/Collins, 1964), Book Two, Ch. XXXI, 211-12.

Getting Rich Off A Woman's Right to Choose Life

By Carol N. Everett

After the anesthetist put her to sleep, I placed my hand on Jenny's abdomen. I felt movement—one of the only babies I can remember moving inside the mother during an abortion. Dr. Johnson proceeded as normal. He cleaned off her cervix with beta-dyne, dilated her cervix, and suctioned briefly to break the bag of amniotic fluid surrounding the baby. The baby did not move after he finished suctioning.

The next step required that the doctor crush the baby inside Jenny's uterus and then remove its body piece by piece using the Bierhof forceps. The first time my favorite abortionist reached in he pulled out placental tissue. The second time he reached in he pulled out the lining around the colon. Immediately I saw the shock on Harvey's (Dr. Johnson) face. I could not see what he pulled out, but the look on his face told me it was serious. His face was ashen as he spoke: "It's over! That's omenum (the term for the viscera connecting the abdominal structures)." He frantically tried to push the bowel back into the uterine cavity, but to no avail. "We have to take her to the hospital, Carol."

"It can't be over," I objected. "The baby is not even dead. It is still intact. We can't take this woman to the hospital with a live baby inside her. It can't be over! Surely there is something we can do!" I know my voice sounded hysterical, but I could not believe this was happening.

"No, Carol, there isn't anything." Harvey pushed back from the table. He leaned toward me, looking dejected, and said quietly, "We *have* to take her to the hospital." Harvey knew he had blown this one badly. He was scared to death, and it showed.

"Where will we take her?" I asked. Garland Memorial was out of the question. Lately we had taken too many botched abortions there. One of the doctors at the hospital was now checking every one of Dr. Johnson's charts, trying to catch one of his travesties.

Harvey stood up, picked up the stainless steel pan for the body parts, and walked out of the room. I followed him into central supply, where he slowly removed his gloves. I silently waited for his decision.

As we headed to his office he said, "I'm going to call Dr. Lloyd; he'll help us." Harvey seemed to always have a list of people who owed him a favor. He called them in at times like this.

My mind raced ahead, clicking off what I knew of medical procedures. If her bowel has come out through the vagina, the uterus has to be perforated. With the baby alive and a bowel resection needed, this will be quite a surgical procedure, requiring several specialists. Dr. Johnson could not do the bowel resection, and what will they do with the baby's body in a hospital?

By now, supervisors and employees were becoming accustomed to the quiet, frantic relocation of a botched abortion to a hospital. They ignored us as best they could.

I checked again with Harvey to be sure everything was set with Lloyd. "What are we going to do?" I asked him.

"Let me think about this," he mumbled. Harvey made some more telephone calls and then finally said, "Move her to your car. Take her to Garland Humana Hospital. They have been trying to get me to use their hospital. Take her to the emergency room entrance, and Dr. Lloyd will meet you there."

He dropped his hand on my shoulder and looked directly into my eyes. "Do not tell anyone what happened. I told Lloyd I was taking care of another doctor's problem. Don't even mention my name," he emphasized.

"Don't worry. I won't." I hurried to the back.

"Leslie, put Jenny in my car." Leslie had helped me move women before, so she knew exactly what to do. She placed the wheelchair next to the operating table and locked the brakes in place.

"Jenny, can you sit up? We are going to move you now."

"Is it over, Carol?" Jenny muttered.

"Jenny, there has been a problem. We have to move you to the hospital for additional surgery. We cannot do it in the clinic." I was calm and matter-of-fact.

"I can't go to the hospital! I don't have any insurance!"

"We have to take you to the hospital. You must be treated. We can't stop now."

"What about money?"

"Jenny, I can't answer you. Help us get you into the wheelchair and out to the car. Is there anyone you would like for us to call to have with you at the hospital?"

"Yes, call Sharon. Tell her what happened. See if she can come to the hospital." As we wheeled Jenny out the back door, she asked, "Are you taking me to the hospital in a car?" She sounded confused.

I took over. "Yes, and Kelley is going to ride with us. Leslie and I will lift your arms while you stand up. I hope it does not hurt, but we have to move you to the car."

Kelley held the IV, her eyes wide. She had never seen anything like this.

I started snapping out orders. "Jenny, I am going to recline that seat as far as I can. Kelley, I will hold the IV while you go around and get in the back seat." Obediently, Kelley hurried around the car and got in. "Here, Kelley, hold it up over her head; keep it running."

"Which hospital are we going to?" Jenny wanted to know.

"Garland Humana."

"I've never heard of that. Where is it?"

"It's a good hospital in Garland. My son had an operation there."

"It hurts! Where's Dr. Johnson?"

"He'll meet us at the hospital."

"How much longer? I can't stand the pain! Hurry! Why is this taking so long?"

"We're going to a good hospital, with the best doctors. It's in Garland and it takes a little longer to get there. You'll be well cared for. It will only be a few more minutes." I tried to keep as calm as possible, much calmer than I actually felt.

Jenny screamed in pain all the way to the hospital. Every time I looked at my daughter I wished that I had not brought her. Kelley was scared, nervous, and stunned.

For some time I had wanted Kelley's validation of abortion and my part in it, but she had been noncommittal. I felt she was acting the part of a pro-choice supporter just to win my approval. If Kelley was going to be good in this business, she had to learn it all. I had recently forced her to watch a big procedure—her first. She did not like it at all. She kept trying to get out of the room. I insisted she stay through the entire procedure, however, and afterwards she was very upset, refusing to talk to me about it. Now this plan was backfiring on me, too. Kelley seemed to be putting herself in Jenny's place. She did not seem at all confident about what her mother was doing.

Riding to the hospital, I too began to identify Jenny with Kelley. This could be my daughter Kelley in trouble. How would I feel if this were happening to my daughter? I did not like the answer.

"Kelley, how's that IV doing?" Back to reality.

"It's still running."

"Good! Thank you, baby, for helping me!" I concentrated on driving and was very relieved when the entrance to Garland Humana appeared ahead. "Jenny, here we are! Let's find the emergency room. There it is!"

I pulled into the parking spot reserved for ambulances and jumped out of the car.

"Kelley, I'm going to get a stretcher. Stay in the car."

A nurse stepped out in the hall as I entered. "May I help you?"

"Yes, I have an emergency admission in my car. We need a gurney."

"Does the patient have a doctor?" she asked as she rounded a corner to get the stretcher.

"Yes, Dr. Lloyd is supposed to meet us here."

An angry Dr. Lloyd came out of nowhere. "Carol, come here! I will tell you right now I am not covering up for Harvey this time!"

The nurse returned with the gurney and Jenny was quickly moved into a room. Suddenly the nurse yelled, "There's Pitocin in the IV! Is she an abortion patient?"

Jenny screamed, "Where is Dr. Johnson?"

"Did Harvey do her abortion, Carol?" Dr. Lloyd questioned.

Before I could answer, Dr. Johnson walked up, slipped his arm over Dr. Lloyd's shoulder, and the two walked toward Jenny's emergency room. Dr. Lloyd was arguing, but I could tell Harvey would win him over, as usual.

I hugged Kelley and sent her back to the clinic in my car.

Dr. Johnson reappeared briefly to direct me to the doctor's lounge to wait while Jenny's surgery was performed. I went through hell in that room while I waited for Harvey. Painful as it was to admit, I knew we were not helping women have a safe abortion. Instead, we were maiming and even killing women. How did this happen? Why did it bother me so much, so suddenly? Why was Jenny's botched abortion making me question my future in the abortion industry? I finally decided it had to do with the look in my daughter's eyes—how she stared at me in the rearview mirror as we drove Jenny to the hospital, the way she looked at me in the hospital when she said, "I want to go! I want to go back to the office!" She had looked right through me. What was it about that look?

Suddenly all of my efforts to convince Kelley we were helping women were revealed for the lies they were, lies to justify myself; and Kelley knew. Kelley saw more than she needed to see. I had made a big mistake in having her go to the hospital with me. Fear of Kelley's rejection engulfed me.

In the doctor's lounge the waiting seemed like an eternity. A million thoughts ran through my mind—my daughter Kelley, Jenny, Harvey, botched abortions, the business. Finally Harvey appeared in the door looking haggard.

"Carol, we don't have a problem anymore."

I couldn't believe my ears. How could we not have a problem? We had really blown it on Jenny. I assumed we would be facing a major lawsuit this time.

"I'll tell you about it later," Harvey said. "Let's get out of here! Did any of her family come?" As we walked out of the hospital I realized I did not feel the usual pride walking with Harvey.

We drove to Harvey's house to pick up Freddie before they drove me home. On the way, he commented, "I have to talk to Dale, the pathologist, in the morning to work out a few things, but I'm sure the abdominal pregnancy was the cause of the colostomy."

I kept my mouth shut, but I certainly talked to myself. "Abdominal pregnancy? That was not an abdominal pregnancy! You examined her before the abortion. You would surely have picked that up in a physical examination of a five-and-a-half-month pregnancy. No competent doctor would ever have started an abortion on a woman with an advanced abdominal pregnancy! So this is how you choose to cover this one up! Have all the doctors who operated with you agreed to write up the records as an abdominal pregnancy? Will the pathologist write up his records the same way? You are going to lie to keep us from being sued, and all of your doctor buddies are going to support your lie!"

I couldn't stand it any longer. "Harvey, we have just ruined a young woman's body and her life! Jenny has had a colostomy! What if she were one of *our* children? What if she were Kelley, or your daughter Jan? How would we feel?"

Harvey ignored my question. He calmly continued with the details of the surgical procedure. "I wrapped the baby in a disposable sheet and threw it in with the trash in the surgical suite. No one will think it is anything other than a disposable sheet."

You really covered your tracks, I thought.

"Lloyd thinks he can resection the colostomy in about six months, so the colostomy will not be permanent," he told me. Thank heaven! Jenny is such a beautiful young woman.

"The hospital administrator at Humana has been trying to get me to move my surgery over there for some time. I'll go see him in the morning. Maybe I can get him to write off the bill," Harvey added.

"Do you think he will?" I asked.

"They need the business, and I will do a few cases over there if they do."

We pulled up to Harvey's house and Freddie joined us. "How did it go?" she asked when she got into the car.

"Everything's all right," he answered. "She had to have a colostomy, but Dr. Smith checked her urinary tract and everything is OK. It was an abdominal pregnancy."

I screamed inside. *He's lying to us–Freddie and me, the people who protect him from anything and everything. He can't even tell us the truth–that* he *blew it!*

I couldn't stand it! I had to let Harvey know I knew he was lying. My hand had been on that baby, and it was perfectly in place inside her uterus.

"Are you going to change the records at the clinic to reflect an abdominal pregnancy?" I asked manipulatively.

"Do you mean it wasn't an abdominal pregnancy?" Freddie shot back, looking first at me, then at Harvey.

On the hot seat, Harvey did not answer directly, but said tersely to me, "You will need to pull that chart and keep it in your office. I'll make some notes about the surgical procedure the next time I'm in the clinic."

"Harvey, what happened?" Freddie demanded.

"Everything's all right, Freddie. Jenny has had an abdominal pregnancy. That's all. It's always critical when we hospitalize a patient from the clinic. You know that."

As we turned the corner of Marsh Lane and headed toward my house, I knew what I had to do about Harvey and his blown procedures. In the future I would make sure Harvey Johnson did not do any abortion past fifteen weeks, which clearly seemed to be his safety zone. I did not know exactly how I was going to accomplish this without Freddie's knowledge, but Harvey Johnson was not going to do another big abortion if I could help it—and I could help it.

I was involved in the abortion industry for six years in the Dallas-Fort Worth, Texas, area. I was ultimately responsible for 35,000 abortions, the death of one woman, the maiming of nineteen others to the point of a hysterectomy or colostomy—I was indeed the Scarlet Lady.

I think of myself now as the Scarlet Lady, but it's different. It's the redemptive blood of Jesus Christ.

Physicians and doctors save lives; abortionists destroy lives. These same complications are taking place across our nation today. In 1992 we know of the deaths of two women from abortion that did not show abortion or any relation to abortion on the death certificate. These deaths will not be recorded at the Centers for Disease Control in Atlanta as abortion deaths. Statistics are slanted; the public never hears the truth, because you see, the family does not want to come forward. They do not want to shed any more disparaging light on their family member. We do not know how many women actually die or are maimed by abortion.

Another common practice of the abortion clinics is doing abortions on women who are not pregnant. This was well documented at our clinics in 1983 by the CBS affiliate Channel 4 in Dallas, and also the Chicago *Sun Times* documented it very well.

How do you do an abortion on a woman who isn't pregnant? This young woman is frightened, so it's a little different sales technique. You say to her, "This pregnancy test is not sensitive enough to pick up a very early pregnancy. You could still be pregnant, and this test would not show it. I *know* you want to know today, don't you? Why don't we do this other test while you are here?" Then we would take her back to the sonogram. You and I know that a sonogram looks at a woman's abdomen and everything in there shows up, pregnant or not. We would just get a shadow on that screen, turn that screen around, and say, " See there? There it is. You are pregnant."

This young woman did not know a pregnant sonogram from a negative sonogram. This is the expert saying, "There it is. You are pregnant." The next question, as you reach out and touch her arm, is, "Do you have your money? Can you do it today?" And far too many of those young women walk right up front.

So how do you do an abortion on that woman? In order for the abortionist to collect his commission, he must have a specimen. So he simply scrapes out more of the lining of the uterus of the young woman who is not pregnant.

I know we have had infertility around since Old Testament days, but have you ever thought about the new high rate of infertility we are seeing today? Have you ever asked yourself how that fits into the abortion picture? We do not have good statistics. Abortion has only been legal twenty years—and anyway, that study would not help sell abortions.

I want to tell you about the way we sold abortions. I know you are going to say, "Carol, we should not be talking about this—sex education, I mean, come on!" But I want you to know that we had a plan, and it started in kindergarten, because we knew that sex education sold abortions. And today, across this nation, abortionists have a plan for comprehensive sex education. They want to get our children earlier and earlier.

Now in kindergarten—I did not actually do this, but I knew this was part of the plan—we would put them boy-girl-boy-girl. Of course in kindergarten these children are not very interested in sex, but we would talk to them about what their mother called their "private parts." We would say to them, "What does your mother say to call your 'private parts'?" They would tell us, and we would laugh. We then would go to a second child with the same question. They would tell us, and again we would laugh. A couple of the kids would pick up on the idea that they were supposed to laugh too. By the time we put the question to the third child and they responded, every child in the classroom laughed. You see, we had well established that their parents did not know what their private parts were. *We* were the experts about sex.

Then we would say, "Boys, this is what you have, and girls, this is what you have. And don't be ashamed of your private parts!" Of course there is not a kindergartner in the world who is ashamed of anything. They would get out on the playground and she would show him hers and he would show her his. We would have accomplished two things. First, they were persuaded that their parents knew nothing about sex or their sexual organs. Second, we had started to break down that natural modesty.

In first, second, and third grade the subject was intercourse, but you know these children are not too interested in intercourse. We had little books, with six- and seven-year-old bodies, nude. Diagrams were there to show them how to have sex, just in case they were interested. This was a book that never went home. They were not allowed to take this book home, but they could look at this book in class anytime they wanted to.

In the fourth grade the subject was masturbation—all alone until you are comfortable, and then in groups of four or five of the same sex. And you tell me that's not that "acceptable alternate lifestyle," homosexuality?

In the fifth grade I came in. I would say to them, "Your mother is an old fuddy-duddy about sex, isn't she?" They would sort of sit there, not sure what I was talking about. "Your mother tells you to save yourself for that special person, doesn't she?" Every mother said that at some time. "Do you think your mother would help you if you decided to become sexually active?" Of course their answer was "No," but I would say, "Don't worry about it. Come to me!"

I knew full well that the next day my telephone would start ringing. They could not drive, but their sister or brother or a friend's brother would bring them in. We would give them a low-dose pill with a high rate of pregnancy. Yes, we gave them a birth control pill we knew they would get pregnant on. The low-dose pill we gave them had to be taken at the same time every day in order to provide protection, but there is not a teenager in the world that does anything at the same time every day. Their mother would nag them to clean their room, nag them to go to school, nag them to finish their homework. Of course their mother did not nag them to take that birth control pill, because she did not know about it.

We could look at the Planned Parenthood statistics, and we could tell that when they were put on any method of contraception their sexual activity would go from zero to five to seven times a week. Then we could achieve our agenda of three to five abortions between the ages of thirteen and eighteen. (The most I ever saw a young woman have was nine abortions, but I have been out of the industry for almost ten years.)

Today there is almost a 50 percent repeat rate. You see, it *is* a method of birth control. The average woman having an abortion today will be twenty-five years of age, but she clearly had her first abortion as a teen—and continues to use it.

Abortionists have an agenda. They have a plan. We react.

In Lake Highlands High School, in Dallas, Texas, they went in the class of my best friend's sixteen-year-old daughter. They had a color movie—pornography—a heterosexual, a homosexual, a handicapped, and an elderly couple having intercourse. When the kids protested, they said, "What's wrong? Don't you want to know how to do it right?" At the end of that class, every child in that class had to put a condom on a banana before they could leave the classroom. The next day the parents poured in, but those pornographic images were set in those little minds. A feeding frenzy took off in that school, and in every class all they talked about was sex, sex, sex—comprehensive sex education.

Now my friend's daughter is pregnant. So who is she going to call? Her friends at the abortion clinic. After all, when she left they gave her a card that said, "We can help you. If you have any questions, give us a call. We have a 24-hour answering service. We are here for you." She calls that number, not understanding the telephone will be answered by a telemarketer, skillfully trained to sell her product.

Have you ever heard a pro-choicer talk about anything but abortion, abortion, abortion? They don't have any choices. We just sold one product, and we sold it well. Actually we had a script in front of every counselor, a script designed to overcome all objections. That's all sales is about, isn't it? Overcome the objection and you get the order, or in this case, you get the abortion.

This young woman will confess to this so-called counselor, "I think I may be pregnant." The counselor will reply, "We can take care of your problem. No one needs to know. What was the date of the first day of your last normal period?" The young woman will figure that date, give it to the so-called counselor, who puts it on a wheel that is actually designed to calculate the birthdate of the baby. But she does not talk about birthdate or baby. She says, "You are eight weeks pregnant."

What did she do? She confirmed this young woman's very worst fear—"I'm pregnant!" You would think she would say, "How in the world can you tell me that over the telephone?" But she is talking to the "expert," and in this frightened young woman's mind, she accepts what the "expert" tells her. The first seed in this long marketing thread is planted. The next question is, "Is this good news or bad news?" What a terrible joke! If it were good news, she would not be calling an abortion clinic. It's bad news, and when she acknowledges that the counselor moves right in: "We can take care of your problem. No one needs to know."

Now the counselor is looking for the fear. Why the fear? To use it to reaffirm the abortion decision anytime this young woman starts to move away. So she starts with "Your parents don't have to know."

That just makes me sick, because I knew that was the easiest sell. They had trusted their parents explicitly for sixteen years, and suddenly some outsider says, "Your parents would kill you," and they believe her. This child cannot sign to have her own ears pierced. She cannot sign to take an aspirin at school. But she can sign for her own abortion.

The thing that makes me most angry is my dog. Every time I take that dog to the veterinarian, I have to sign for her to have surgery. I have to sign for everything they do to that dog. And the veterinary clinics of my state are regularly inspected by the health department, but the abortion clinics are not. We *do* take better care of the animals of this nation than we do our women!

Now the counselor has identified the fear. She has her sales pitch anytime the client moves away. So she goes to the next question: "Does the father know?" Why in the world is this poor guy hung out here as the father? The mother's not a mother, and the baby's not a baby, but here he is a father? What are they saying? They are saying, "Take your guilt and your anger and blame him. It's his fault!" All the way through the abortion clinic you will hear, "Did the father come with you? Did the father give you money?" That is precisely why 75 percent of these relationships break up ninety days after the abortion—as my own marriage did. Worse than that, it's that wedge in God-ordained relationships between men and women. I'm not even certain that we, the church, yet understand that abortion is designed to break down God's institution of the family.

My abortion was twenty years ago—February 16. These last couple of years have been very difficult. My two adult children have been dealing with the fact that they lost a sister. This is the first year that we have really been able to all cry together on the anniversary of her death.

"It's $250. Don't panic! Wait a minute! You are not thinking logically. Do you have a checking account or a savings account? Or do you have a Mastercard or Visa or American Express card?" Yes, check with your bank card companies, because they alone determine if abortions are allowed to be charged. American Express not only allows abortions to be charged, but the company supports Planned Parenthood, the largest abortion provider in the nation.

"No money? OK, this is what you need to do. Go to all your friends and borrow $5, $10, or $25. Get yourself a part-time job. You know you can pay them back in six months or a year."

I still have that vivid picture of that young woman coming in the front door with this big bag of coins. She did not have a dollar bill in there! All I could think about was how long it was going to take *me* to count that money, so I made her count it out in dollars, starting with the quarters. She was three cents short. I would not have lost her for three cents. This young man sitting in the reception area did not know that, though. He jumped up, slammed three cents on the counter, and said, "Here's the money. Do her abortion!"

If abortions are so good for women, why aren't they free? It's because this is the largest unregulated legal industry in our nation today.

For the first sixteen years after *Roe v. Wade*, public perception was that abortion came under the same ethical standards as all other branches of medicine. The reality is that states failed to regulate this new abortion industry. In July, 1989, the *Webster v. Reproductive Health Services* case out of Missouri gave us the first minor regulations of the abortion clinic. The court let stand the statutory preamble: tests for viability at twenty weeks gestation, comprehensive restriction of the use of public funding, public employees, and public facilities to perform and assist in abortions. But also in this case the Supreme Court invited states to address the abortion industry.

In the 1989-90 session, some forty-two states addressed the abortion issue. No real regulation came out of that because the only one that made it through with anything strong was Pennsylvania. On June 29, 1992, the Supreme Court announced their opinion in the *Planned Parenthood of Southeastern Pennsylvania v. Robert P. Casey* case. This decision offered the first regulation limiting the abortion issue with informed consent, a 24-hour waiting period prior to the performance of an abortion, parental informed consent, and the medical emergency definition used in the statute. Now in Pennsylvania—and only Mississippi has followed suit—can a woman be told the truth about what is being removed. There is something about telling a woman it's a choice, yet not being able to tell her the truth about fetal development, that cheapens a woman.

Abortion is the most commonly performed surgical procedure in the United States today (excluding circumcision). Abortion is the only surgical procedure performed without an informed consent except in those two states of Pennsylvania and Mississippi. Abortion is not about rights or choices, or even rape or incest. Abortion is about money. It is a skillfully marketed product, sold to a frightened young woman at a crisis time in her life. She buys that product, finds it defective, but she can't return it for a refund. Her baby is dead.

I worked on a straight commission, too. Twenty-five dollars does not sound like a lot of money, but the last month we did 545 abortion, so 545 times $25 will tell you my last month's income was $13,625—and that was a bad month!

The abortionist works on a straight commission. He is paid a percentage, and the abortion industry is legal through all nine months of pregnancy. Some people are convinced that is not true. They say that *Roe v. Wade* just talked about the first three months of pregnancy. What you do not hear is that *Doe v. Bolton,* the companion case of *Roe,* heard the very same day, did address this broader issue. It said that for the "health of the mother" an abortion could be completed through all nine months of pregnancy. Of course we knew that encompassed mental health, so we would say to this frightened young woman, "You would have problems with this pregnancy should you carry it to term?" She would say "Yes" and we would chart it "emotional health." The biggest baby I ever personally helped abort was thirty-two weeks. That baby clearly could have lived outside its mother's uterus.

Abortions cost roughly from $250 to $8,000. That higher-end figure is clearly a third-trimester abortion, advertised in the *LA Times.* For that third trimester, or even a second-trimester abortion, the abortionist puts 50 percent of the fee in his pocket. He can do three of those an hour, so that's $12,000 an hour. We all know that the majority of abortions are clearly first-trimester abortions—about 95 percent. For that $250 abortion he can't make that much money, can he? He makes a third of the fee, a minimum of $75 in this nation. We had a technique to keep our abortionist doing ten to twelve abortions an hour. You see, we had two teams of two women that worked with each abortionist. Team number one would set up girl number one, and the abortionist would go in and do that abortion, while across the hall team number two would set up girl number two. When the abortionist finished abortion number one he would run across the hall to do abortion number two. Meanwhile, team number one had to get the first girl out, clean the room, and get girl number three set up so that when he finished abortion number two he could run across the hall and do abortion number three. Using that technique, we could keep them all doing ten to twelve an hour. Ten times $75 is $750 an hour; twelve times $75 is $900 an hour. I heard an abortionist testify under oath in San Diego in a court of law that he worked eighteen hours a week, did 150 abortions a week. According to my math, the minimum that abortionist could make is $45,000 a month. That man testified he was paid in cash at the end of the day—no Form 1099, no W-2 form. That's what abortion is about! A part-time job, working 18 hours a week, making $45,000 a month cash—I'm sure they reported all of that to the IRS!

I wanted to be a millionaire. It's pretty simple: twenty-five into a million says I only needed to do 40,000 abortions a year, and I planned to do it! But we had some problems. We had two abortion clinics going fairly smoothly, but we could not do 40,000 abortions out of them. I worked my plan and planned my work on that side. I had a $250,000 yellow-page advertising budget in place. I just needed to open three abortion clinics in 1983, then I could be a millionaire in 1984. We were having so many internal problems, however, that I had to have some help. I called in a business counselor who said he could solve our problems in thirty days. I asked him how much he was going to charge us; he said, "I'll solve your problem by meeting with each of you for an hour a week for the next four weeks." I said, "Sold!" I would pay him *any* amount of money.

It's a very long story, but this counselor happened to be a pastor, a pastor who laid out the plan of salvation to me. He said that God had allowed him to be in that situation for thirty days. Just twenty-seven days after he came in, my prayer of "Lord, if this isn't where you want me, hit me over the head with a two-by-four" was answered.

That two-by-four was the CBS affiliate doing an exposé on abortion clinics doing abortions on women who were not pregnant. They caught us red-handed, and I knew that I was not to be in the abortion industry. They showed clearly that we were doing abortions on women who were not pregnant, and we were using a man to do abortions who was not a licensed physician. This was perfectly legal in the state of Texas. Do you know what happened as a result of the TV report? Nothing! On the third day I went back to collect my personal belongings, and what I saw turned even *my* stomach. That terrible "advertisement" had been good for business. People were standing in line to get in the front door. They were lined up down the hall. Not one city, state, or federal authority was investigating us. What we were doing to those women was perfectly legal, because the industry is not regulated.

I was not instantly pro-life. I was a hurting, angry, baby-killing, woman-killing woman. The man who led me to Christ and his wife spent some part of every day with me for eighteen months.

They were not just being nice to me; they were feeding me Scripture. They were answering every question with the Word of God. I would say, "I'm scared," and they would say, "God . . . [didn't give] us the spirit of fear; but of power, and of love, and a sound mind" (2 Tim. 1:7, KJV). I started to like that. And I found Psalm 139.

As I read how each of us is fearfully and wonderfully made, how we are knitted together inside the darkness of our mother's womb, I knew I had been involved in the murder of 35,000 babies. And that was a heaviness. I did not find the word *abortion* anywhere in that Bible, either. I just knew I could not be forgiven. Then I found 1 John 1:9, and I read that if you will repent and confess your sins "He is faithful and just to forgive." I started confessing and repenting of one and tens and thousands. I'm now almost a ten-year-old Christian, and He is not through with me yet!

There have been days in my life when people have been in my face and said, "How do you think you can be forgiven, lady? You've killed 35,000 babies! You can't get to heaven!" I have to remember that's where they are, but I also know that Psalm 103:12 says that our sins are "as far as the east is from the west." Today I really believe that my call may well be to keep telling this story because our church needs to know. I think we have made some mistakes in the pro-life movement. We have been trying to educate the world, and the world is not going to have the morals to make the difference. It's the church of Jesus Christ that will make the difference.

I know that my church is hurting. Every time I go into a church, someone will squeeze my hand—sometimes even a deacon's wife—and say, "I know what you are talking about, but I can't tell anyone." *Newsweek* reported in May 1989 that one out of six women sitting in our church pews has had an abortion. And there is a man for every woman. The men are just starting to come forward. Last October, *USA Today* released a report that showed that 70 percent of the people who walked through the doors of the abortion clinic will say they are churched, will say they are Christians at some level. And 27 percent of those will say they have been in church once a week. We in the church need the truth.

As a Southern Baptist, I want to help our people combat this destructive force. As a post-aborted mother, I implore all Christians to address this issue to advance the healing process in our churches. When the church reaches out in love and forgiveness, we who have experienced abortion—both men and women—can confess, repent, and start to understand that the forgiving blood of Christ covers even an abortion. I am convinced that our nation is a mission field of pain from abortion and sexual activity outside of God's plan.

There are over three thousand crisis pregnancy centers across this nation, ministering to the needs of those young women. Of course you never read it in the paper or hear it on the news, because it is not considered newsworthy. They never charge those young women money. If you hear anything about them, they are called "fake abortion clinics" because last year we saved 300,000 babies across this nation. If you just multiply 300,000 times $200, we cost the abortion industry $60 million last year.

Young women walk through the doors of those crisis pregnancy centers, not understanding that they are going to hear the gospel in there. Although not all of these centers share the gospel, about 15 percent of those young women who walk through the doors pray to receive Jesus Christ as their personal Savior. That is ultimately our answer. I believe this is the mission field that is going to be the one that changes the hearts of our nation.

RU-486
Another Method of
Abortion

By J. C. Willke

RU-486 is the well-known French abortion pill. Before discussing it, let us first review female physiology a bit.

There are two female hormones. One is estrogen. When this hormone is produced, the girl's body turns into a woman's. It shapes her body and develops her breasts. When this hormone leaves, she goes through "change of life." It is one of the two reproductive hormones.

The second hormone is progesterone, sometimes called the pregnancy hormone. It is produced in a cyclic fashion in the second half of every month. Not much is produced in the first half of her menstrual month, then there is a substantial amount of it produced. The function of this hormone is to thicken and prepare the lining of the womb for the nesting of a new embryo. If she is pregnant that month, production of this hormone increases markedly and is maintained throughout the pregnancy. It can properly be called a nutritive hormone. If she does not get pregnant that month, then this hormone is withdrawn and the lining of the womb sloughs in what is known as menstruation.

RU-486 blocks the action of progesterone. Its essential action could be compared to a grape on the vine. If you were to pinch the stem so as to prevent the nutritive sap from getting to the grape, then the grape would wither, die, and drop off. Essentially, this is what is done when this pill functions to end a pregnancy. It deprives the developing embryonic baby of this vital nutrient hormone, progesterone, and so this tiny one withers, dies, and is lost, along with the lining of the womb, which is not maintained because of the blocking of this hormone.

It is important to emphasize that there is only one scientifically proven function for this pill and that is to kill a developing baby after his or her heart has begun to beat. This pill is not a contraceptive. It does not prevent the release of the fertilized ovum. This pill may also have a function as a morning-after pill, although experiments continue on this. Nothing has yet been proven. It has been tried as a once-a-month pill and has been found to be ineffective and totally rejected by the women on whom it was tried. I'll discuss its potential therapeutic functions, but it is important to repeat there is only one proven function for this pill, and that is to destroy the life of an embryonic baby—after his or her heart has begun to beat.

There is only a short window in time during which this pill is effective in destroying an embryonic baby. If we count from the first day of the last normal menstrual period, four weeks have elapsed when her period is due. The fifth week, she does not yet go to a doctor, as she could simply be late for her period. The earliest a woman goes to the doctor is at the end of that fifth week. This pill works only in the sixth and seventh weeks. After that it becomes progressively more ineffective. In France, it is only given in those first seven weeks, which means, only during that two-week window. In the United Kingdom, it is being given in the first nine weeks. Translated, that means a four-week window in time. There is substantial evidence to indicate, however, that the further into pregnancy, the less effective the pill becomes.

In those first few weeks, if she is pregnant and if everything else is in order, studies have shown that if Ru-486 is used alone, from 60 to 80 percent of the time it will be effective in killing that embryo and ending the pregnancy. This is not effective enough for the pill to be used as a major drug on the open market. Therefore, it is almost always followed by a second drug. Prostaglandin is a hormone that produces violent contractions of the uterus. It produces violent labor and delivery of whatever size baby she carries. Accordingly, most of the time prostaglandin is added after the pills have been taken. When used together these achieve a 95 percent success rate.

There still remain however, five, some say eight or ten percent of the women who still do not abort. The answer by the abortion folks is that she must then have a surgical scraping out of her womb, a surgical abortion, for if she carries that surviving baby to term, there is a substantial risk of fetal deformity.

Let me take you through the clinical routine that has been established in France for the use of this pill. It is a very tightly controlled clinical situation, quite unlike medical practice in an open clinical setting, such as one would find in most nations. But let's be that woman who goes to the clinic in France and wants to use this pill.

First, her history is taken. A complete physical examination is done, plus a pregnancy test. Assuming her pregnancy is confirmed and it is that window of time, a complete blood count is done. If she is anemic the pill is not used. Then she is asked a series of questions; if she has any of the following problems she will not get the drug. Is she a smoker? Sorry, no pill. Does she have circulation problems, asthma, high blood pressure, fibroid tumors on the uterus, glaucoma (that is increased pressure in the eye), stomach ulcers, colitis (inflammation of the bowel)? Does she have infection of the female organs? Has she had a recent caesarean section? If she says yes to any of these, she is not given the pill. Finally, it is usual to give an ultrasonic exam to confirm that her pregnancy is not too far advanced for the pill to work.

She then is given a paper to sign. This is a legal release form and is very interesting because of one section. This section says that she agrees to take the pill, and then the prostaglandin drug, and if she does not abort, she will then submit to a surgical abortion. It states that if she fails to abort from the drugs, but then refuses to have a surgical abortion and goes on to have her baby, if the baby is deformed, she will not enter into a lawsuit against the company.

French law requires a waiting period of one week. She then returns to the clinic, swallows the pills in the presence of the doctor, and departs. She returns for a third visit. If she has passed baby parts she must collect those parts in a jar and bring them to the clinic for examination. If she has not aborted, she is then given the prostaglandin drug and kept in the clinic for the balance of the day. If she has not aborted by late afternoon, she is taken into the operating room and a surgical abortion is done. She is sent home.

She returns for the fourth visit and has a physical exam. If all is well, this may be her last visit. But it very commonly is not, for a variety of reasons. The major reason for additional return visits is continued, prolonged, and heavy bleeding. Typically, she will bleed from ten to as long as forty days. In the largest study out of the United States, published in *The New England Journal of Medicine,* one woman in every one hundred bled so long and so much that she needed to have her womb scraped out to stop the bleeding.[1] In the most recent large study, in the United Kingdom, one woman in every one hundred needed a blood transfusion.[2]

Other problems? Yes. Pain. Pain was a constant major problem for women, with one in four needing narcotic injections for the pain. Nausea and vomiting are also a constant pattern.

But the big one is death from heart attacks. The French company has admitted that one woman died from a heart attack after having had these drugs. It also admits to two other near-deaths. One of these was a cardiac arrest, the other was a ventricular fibrillation. The answer to cardiac arrest is to start the heart again. The only way to do that is with electric shock, with a machine called a defibrillator. It so happens that this woman's heart stopped while she was in a clinic equipped with this very technical piece of equipment. They shocked her, started her heart again and she lives. But, if she had been anywhere but that clinic, she'd be dead. The second woman had a ventricular fibrillation, which is a rhythm disturbance of the heart in which the heart stops pumping and the muscle just quivers. That is quickly fatal unless the proper rhythm is restored. The only way to restore it is by electric shock by a defibrillator. Fortunately for both of these women, they were in a technically equipped clinic. If they had been anywhere else they would have been dead. We know of a fourth that was not reported in the literature. These were out of the first 80,000 abortions done in France. If we assume that the two women would have died anywhere else, and we have that fourth death, then we have four deaths in 80,000. If that record maintains, there will be five deaths in 100,000. That compares to one or two deaths reported for every 100,000 suction abortions.

Now let's look at the psychological aspects of this. We know that a significant number of all women who have surgical abortions are extremely ambivalent about the abortion decision. They really don't want to do this. Something deep inside of them fights against it. And yet, they feel they have no other option. They feel they are boxed in so they go ahead and have the abortion. A psychological defense mechanism here is for her to close her eyes while she is on the operating table and say, "I don't want this, I don't want this. They are forcing it on me, they are doing it to me." That won't work with the pill, for now she herself swallows the pills. *She* did it, and there is no denying it. If she passes baby parts at home, she sees them and brings the pieces back in. We are of the opinion that there will be just as much post-abortion psychic trauma from taking the pill as we now see from surgical abortion.

Now let's look at the effect this pill has on the baby. There will be women who take the pill who do not abort, change their minds, and go on to deliver. There can be many reasons for this: She herself was very ambivalent. The pill didn't work. She takes it as a sign that it was not meant to be. She goes on to have her baby. Other women will talk with their husband, boyfriend, mother, girl friends, and they will be talked out of going for the surgical abortion. Another lady might not have understood the instructions, and didn't take all the pills, or maybe shared them with her sister. Another dropped one of the pills in the toilet and only took the other one. All of these did not abort. Some will change their minds and carry to term. What will be the result of having these babies?

She has taken a powerful, artificial, poisonous steroid drug. The purpose of this poison was to kill her developing baby. It didn't quite work. But it was poisonous, and it did injure the baby, and, most importantly, it was taken at the time of organogenesis. That is, it was taken at the time when the legs and arms and fingers and heart are being built. It didn't quite kill this little child, but it can cause a malformation. From the malformations that we have seen in animals and in some babies to date, we are led to believe the results will be similar to those seen several decades ago from the drug, thalidomide. This was a drug sold over the counter in Germany for headaches. Pregnant women took it and they delivered babies with grotesque deformities of their arms and legs. It looks like this one may do the same.

Don't forget, there are two drugs here. The second is prostaglandin. Whether one or the other causes trouble will make little difference to the baby. We have one reported case from France of such a child who was born at about 4-1/2 months, dead, with grotesque deformities of its lower extremities. We have reports from Brazil of women who were able to get the prostaglandin alone, took it in early pregnancy and delivered babies with deformities of their skulls.

Whether or not it will do this in many cases, we don't know. It does do it consistently in rabbits. It does not do it in mice. We do have some human babies deformed. I believe that it is imperative for all nations to withhold the use of this drug until enough time has gone by to be sure that it is truly safe for babies.

Now let me turn to the alleged therapeutic uses of this drug. One of the possible uses that has received a lot of publicity is the treatment of a certain type of brain tumor known as meningioma. This is a slow-growing tumor that can exist as long as ten years. It is characterized by stops and starts, that is, it will grow for awhile and then stop for awhile. It does most of its damage by the pressure of the tumor expanding. So, it's a little hard to trace whether or not the medicine you are using is helping. This tumor has what we call progesterone receptors. Theoretically, the use of this pill could lock up those receptors and might retard the growth of the tumor. Well, let's see what's reported. In *The Journal of Neurosurgery* 1991, we find the only major report to date. It is of fourteen patients. In four of these the tumor continued to grow. In five the tumor was unchanged. Five saw a minor decrease in size but later regrowth.[3] Now that's not even a very encouraging report. Certainly, it is not a dramatic one. Remember, these tumors come in both men and women. What were the side effects? In women, onset of menopause and hot flashes, baldness, fatigue. Men all reported growth of their breasts. All in all, this is hardly a miracle drug.

Certain breast cancers also have progesterone receptors. What of treating these? To date there is one report in the literature. It was of twenty-two women, only four of whom had some benefit from the drug, but all four of those had recurrences and died.[4] There are more studies of both of these tumors under way.

Another suggested use for it is for an overproduction of adrenal hormone in a condition called Cushings Syndrome. Here we see another function of this drug. It has antiglucocorticoid activity. By virtue of this function, it should stop and reverse Cushings Syndrome. In fact, reports so far show that the woman's pituitary gland begins to secrete an antidote which blocks the action of this pill. That is the report in *The Annals d'Endocrinologie*.[5]

Now let me quote a few authorities who have reason to know a great deal about this pill. Several years ago it was taken off the market in France. The French Minister of Health personally put it back on the market, and the French government has been paying for its use ever since. Here is a quote from that Health Minister. "The doctor must have immediate access to an electrocardiogram as well as therapeutic equipment for cardiopulmonary resuscitation, a defibrillator, and intravenous injection drugs."[6] The president of the Roussel Uclaf company, Dr. Sakiz, in an article on this concluded with this statement, "The woman must live with this for a full week; this is an appalling psychological ordeal."[7] And here is the medical director of the Planned Parenthood Federation of America, Louise Tyrer, saying, "It is still an abortion and still requires close medical supervision."[8]

The book, *RU-486 Myths*, published by the Massachusetts Institute of Technology with three authors—all three of whom can quite accurately be described as radical pro-abortion feminists—denounces the pill. An honest description of their book would be that they scathingly denounce the pill. Let me outline their interesting reasoning. Their book documents in minute detail the dangers of the pill. It also discusses in detail the fact that this pill has become, almost totally, an object of politics in the United States. The pro-abortion movement sees having this pill legalized in the United States as one of its political goals. The authors tell us that if the drug is licensed, many of the clinics that do surgical abortions will be closed. Then the pill will be used for awhile, but soon it will become evident that the pill is very dangerous to women, and will deform their babies. In due time the United States Food and Drug Administration will take the drug off the market and forbid its use. At such time they fear that the anti-abortion forces in the United States would be able to prevent the reopening of the surgical abortion clinics, and there would be no way for many women in the United States to get abortions. Consequently, they oppose the pill.[9] I would suggest that anyone who really wants some ammunition against the pill should carefully read this book and quote freely from it.

In summary, then, here is where the argument on the pill stands. Those who favor its use say that it is more private, but a surgical abortion takes one visit. Using RU-486 requires three or four. It is not more private. They say it is less expensive, but until you do the various blood tests, ultrasounds, office visits, and pay for both of these medications, this (at least in the United States and United Kingdom) will cost approximately twice as much as a surgical abortion.

They say it is safer than a surgical abortion. I have just told you, in terms of deaths, it is probably more dangerous, and in terms of injury to the mother very likely more so. They say that it is psychologically more benign, but we have good reason to question that. It may or may not be, but it very likely could be even more damaging to a woman's psychological makeup. They say it is quicker, but that is ridiculous. A visit to a surgical abortionist takes a half of one day. This takes several days spread over a week or two.

Now I would like to add a bit of history to this. All of us know of the ugly blot on our civilization of the Nazi holocaust. The name Auschwitz is known to everyone. What many have forgotten is that a huge synthetic rubber plant was built near Auschwitz by slave labor and that 25,000 laborers died in its construction. The company that built it was I. G. Farben. Farben owned a subsidiary company by the name of Degesch. This company developed a poison. The name of this poison was Zyklon-D. It was this poison that was used in the gas chambers in which millions of Jews, Poles, Gypsies, Russian prisoners of war, and others were killed. Zyklon-D made Farben a lot of money during the war. It was truly a human pesticide. After the war, the Allied military government split I. G. Farben into three pieces: BASF, Bayer, and Hoechst A. G.

Let me tell you a little bit about Hoechst. They do $7 billion worth of business in the U.S. every year. They own the Celanese Corporation and Roussel Uclaf; they have a large pharmaceutical company based in New Jersey. They own agricultural chemicals, pesticides, and drugs.

Will the pill come here? Hoechst controls whether or not Roussel Uclaf can or will extend the license. If Hoechst, in Frankfurt, says "no go," the Parisian company cannot send a license. If there is no license, then this drug doesn't come to the U.S.

There is one exception to this. A decade ago an agreement was made with the World Health Organization that Third World countries could use the pill, and if Hoechst and Roussel would not grant the rights, these countries had the right to make it anyway. China is one of those countries that is making and using it. But, in the First World, and that is all of Europe, Canada, the U.S., Japan, Australia, and New Zealand, they cannot bring it in unless the parent company in Frankfurt gives permission for it to come in.

Several years ago, pro-abortion delegations were going to Europe, including Kate Michelman and the National Organization of *Some* Women. In response in December 1990, I led a delegation to Berlin and visited Schering A.G. It makes a prostaglandin. We visited Frankfurt, the home office of Hoechst, and Roussel Uclaf in Paris. We also visited Rhone-Poulenc Rorer in Paris, which makes another prostaglandin. Dr. Richard Land and Dr. Joe McIlhaney were on the team that I led. I did not bring Right to Life people with me, because the companies knew we were opposed to it. So I reached out to para-pro-life groups and churches, and the response was wonderful.

Those who came were the president or his or her representative. We also had: Knights of Columbus; Lutherans for Life; a very strong letter from Dr. Bob Dugan from the National Association of Evangelicals; Phyllis Schlafly of Eagle Forum; a very strong letter from Cardinal O'Connor in New York; American Academy of Medical Ethics (Dr. McIlhaney represented them); Concerned Women for America; a very strong letter from Dr. T. James Kennedy, who spoke for the broadcasting industry; Tom Minnery, vice-president of Focus on the Family; William Sherwin, representing International Right to Life Federation; and Drs. Glasow and Gerster from my office.

In talking to those folks, we never used the word "boycott," but it hung over our discussions like a cloud. Dr. Land explained that Southern Baptists really aren't southern, and how often Southern Baptists go to church. This was to contrast with the typical western European practice of being baptized, married, and buried in church whether you are Anglican, Catholic, Lutheran, or Presbyterian. Three or four percent of the people in England go to church. Dr. Land said, "If this drug comes to America, it will ignite a fire storm." Dr. Jean Garton represented Lutherans for Life. She is the first woman to sit on the ruling Synod of the Lutheran Church, Missouri Synod. She said Missouri Synod Lutherans had never really been too involved in issues like this, "but this pill has galvanized us."

And so, each of our people in turn spoke. Each of our interviews was a full afternoon and done very professionally. We let these companies know that they truly were sitting on a keg of dynamite if they brought that pill to America.

First, they do not want to extend a license unless they have government approval. They have that now. Second, they do not want to extend a license unless there is general public acceptance of abortion. That is why we need to inform them that abortion is not publicly accepted. Third, they do not want to extend a license unless there is a usable prostaglandin, cleared and on the market, for this purpose. Finally, they do not want to extend a license unless there are tight controls and close medical supervision and equipment like defibrillators. If these are satisfied, they will extend the license.

These companies also are worried. They are worried about a

boycott. They should be. They are worried about medical liability. They should be. They are worried about product liability.

Most recently Dr. Sakiz from Roussel Uclaf said he would like to bring RU-486 into this country, but his company does not want its name on the pill.[10] His company wants some other company to ask for the license. In a very professional manner we gave them a strong message.

There is another company involved. It is G.D. Searle, a drug company located just outside Chicago. A few years back, when the FDA voted to approve it, I testified against licensing an oral form of prostaglandin called Cytotecit. It is used with arthritis drugs like aspirin and ibuprofin to prevent your stomach from eroding and bleeding. It is on the market. Considering the liability involved, most doctors probably wouldn't use it for abortion unless its producer went to the FDA and the FDA said yes they could use it for that purpose. The medical liabilities would be profound. Searle has condemned the use of this pill for abortions in Brazil. At that hearing in 1988 when I testified against it, Searle said that they do not want it used for abortion. David Kessler, who was reappointed by Bill Clinton to stay on as FDA head, invited the president of Roussel Uclaf to come to America. Dr. Sakiz met with Kessler and, according to *The New York Times*[11] and a couple of other reports, Kessler made a pitch to Sakiz to bring the pill here and assured him that he would see to it that Searle okayed the use of their prostaglandin, Cytotec. According to all of our information, Searle is extremely reluctant to do this. Searle is owned by Monsanto which makes the sweetener, NutriSweet. That would make a tempting target for us!

So the game is not over. With Searle becoming conscious of the fact that many Americans don't want them to do this, they may not apply for this new use for this pill. And if the German company doesn't give the Parisian company permission to ask for a license, there will be no RU-486 in America.

Now, you might have read that China is going to bring it in. But from all the information we have, the drug from China is identical to RU-486. The international contract said they can use it in China, but can't bring it here.

Obviously the Clinton administration is exerting great pressure from Clinton, but if I could paraphrase something from his campaign, "It's the license, stupid." Zillions of cards need to be sent to the Hoechst Roussel Co. in New Jersey. They should carry a message that we don't want the parent company to extend that license. If we barrage them with enough postcards, we are going to keep that drug out of this country.

Our opponents have told them the Right to Life movement is dead because of the election results. We want to tell Hoechst that we are very much alive and that the church in America has been electrified by this.

An exit poll done by a consortium of the four major networks during the last presidential election—it was called the Voters Research and Survey Poll[12]—has been suppressed. That poll asked the question, "Which one or two issues mattered most in deciding your vote?" Thirteen percent of the entire electorate voted on the issue of abortion. Here are the numbers: Bush got 7.2 percent and Clinton 4.6 percent of those voters. Bush's increment was 2-1/2 votes out of every 100 votes cast because he was pro-life, and Clinton got hurt by that much. There was another choice: "family values." Fifteen percent of people chose that in addition to the 13 percent who chose abortion. How did they vote? Bush 10 percent, Clinton 3-1/2 percent. Add that increment of 6-1/2 to the 2-1/2 and we have 9 points that Bush was up on Clinton, or if you please, that Clinton was down on these values issues. Abortion helped Bush. Abortion hurt Clinton badly.

So much for changing the position of the Republican Party. Here's the big one. "Economy and jobs," 43 percent of people chose it, and Clinton won it 22-10. That's why Clinton won the election. He did not win the election on abortion.

Further, two women selected abortion for every one man. The men who selected abortion went for Bush 65-25. The women voted for Bush 50-42. In the election, Clinton was badly hurt by the abortion and family values issues. The problem was the economy, and it overrode everything else.

We must write and call and tell Hoechst that we are extremely upset. If you are a doctor and that pill comes to this country, tell their agents to just quit calling on you. If you have a Hoechst representative in your congregation, get that person to write the home office and tell them of your concerns.

In 1856 the anti-slavery movement had come a long way. Many thought it had peaked. It was five years before the Civil War. In 1856 there was a critical race for the presidency. James Buchanan was a Democrat and supported slavery. John Fremont, whose party had just taken the name Republican, was charismatic. Everyone thought he had it by a mile. He was against slavery. The race tightened in the stretch, a lot of mud was thrown, Buchanan won. They were faced with four more years of a pro-slavery administration. In early 1857 the Supreme Court brought down the *Dred Scott* decision. *Dred Scott* said, once and for all, that black people were not legal persons. This extended to all of the states. The Court said, don't bring us slavery anymore. It is over. We have settled it. That sounds like the recent *Casey* decision.

Later that year there was a very important race in Illinois. An anti-slavery hero was running for the Senate against a pro-slavery candidate, but Abe Lincoln lost. Talk about depression. But three years later Lincoln was elected president and slavery was doomed.

We each have a role to play in these turbulent times. I sincerely believe that those of us who have been given certain talents have the responsibility to give them back.

When he was barnstorming the country in the late '70s, Francis Schaeffer, a Presbyterian theologian, said, "If we don't begin to use our freedom, to preserve our freedom, we will lose our freedom and our children and grandchildren will not call us blessed."[13]

Endnotes

[1]Silvestre, et al, "Voluntary Interruption of Pregnancy with RU-486 and Prostaglandin," *The New England Journal of Medicine*, Vol. 322, No. 10, 8 March 1990.

[2]"Efficacy and Tolerance of Mifepristone and Prostaglandin in 1st Trimester Abortion," UK Multicentre Trial, *Br. J. OB. Gyn.*, June 1990, Vol. 97, 480-486.

[3]Grunberg, et al, "Treatment of Unresectable Meningiomas with RU-486," *Journal of Neurosurgery*, June 1991, Vol. 74, 861-866.

[4]Romieu, et al, "RU-486 in Advanced Breast Cancer," Bull Cancer, 74 (1987), 455-461.

[5]"L'action Antiglucocorticoide, du RU-486," *Annales d'Endocrinologie*, (Paris) 1989, 50, 208-217.

[6]Directive, J. Girard, Minister of Health and Social Protection, Rep. Francaise, April 12, 1990, Paris.

[7]"Drug Firm Defends Marketing Strategy," *LeMonde* (French), *Guardian Weekly* (English), 19 Aug. 1990, 16.

[8]J. Foreman, "U.S. Proponents Widen Push for Availability," *Boston Globe*, 1 Aug. 1990, 1.

[9]Raymond, et al, "RU-486, Misconceptions, Myths and Morals, published by Institute on Women and Technology, Cambridge, Mass., 1991, ISBN 0-9630083-0-7.

[10]S. Okie, "Pill to be Sold Abroad," *Washington Post,* Health J, 22 May 1990, 7.

[11]"Will It End the Abortion Debate?" *Time,* 14 June 1993, 53.

[12]Voter Research Survey Poll, Exit poll by consortium of 4 major TV networks, Nov. 1992.

[13]Francis Schaeffer, personal communication.

Southern Baptist Heritage of Life

By Timothy George

A Major Omission

The date: March, 1980. The place: the Roosevelt Hotel in New York City. The occasion: the annual seminar of the Christian Life Commission of the Southern Baptist Convention. Some four hundred registrants from twenty-five different states gathered on this occasion at the beginning of a new decade to discuss "Ethical Issues for the Eighties." The speakers addressed a host of concerns which they felt would be on the front burner of the ethical agenda in the decade ahead. Kirby Godsey, president of Mercer University, was there to talk about the crisis in education. Benjamin Hooks addressed the issue of race relations. Barry Commoner spoke about energy. Frances Lappé addressed the question of world hunger. Kurt Waldheim, the sitting secretary-general of the United Nations, talked about the prospects for peace in a world of conflict. There were papers on church-state tensions and personal lifestyle issues. And yes, Sara Weddington, special assistant to President Jimmy Carter, also made an appearance and gave a lively speech on women in the eighties.[1]

Looking back now on this seminar thirteen years later, one is almost thunderstruck by an omission of gargantuan proportions. In a conference intended to delineate the most pressing ethical issues to be faced by the American people in the 1980s, not one single speaker addressed the issue of abortion. Not even Sara Weddington, who had successfully argued the case of *Roe v. Wade* before the Supreme Court seven years before, made any reference to her historic role in this landmark decision. She spoke only in the code language about the eighties being a decade of increasing choice for women.

No one will dispute the urgency of the issues which were discussed on that occasion: racism, the nuclear arms buildup, the energy crisis, and so forth. But how can we account for the total lack of prescience on the part of the planners and participants of this conference that produced a conspiracy of silence on what would prove during the 1980s to be one of the most explosive, unnerving, and divisive moral struggles in the history of the American Republic?

Shifting Perspectives

Looking back now, we can see that at least part of the explanation is related to the fact that the 1980 CLC seminar occurred on the eve of a decade of denominational turbulence in the SBC. While the controversy in the SBC was a complex phenomenon involving serious theological, institutional, and cultural dimensions, it was, especially in its early stages, generated by a widespread reaction of the grass-roots constituency against a denominational bureaucracy from which they felt deep alienation. As evidence of this disjunction, the Southern Baptist Convention, meeting in St. Louis a mere three months after the CLC seminar in New York City, passed a resolution condemning the use of tax money for abortion on demand and calling for a constitutional amendment prohibiting abortion except to save the life of the mother.

There was at least an intuitive awareness of this grass-roots insurgency among some of the participants at the CLC conference in New York. Dr. Jimmy Allen, at that time the immediate past president of the SBC, preached a sermon in which he expressed his concern about the direction of a new and restless activism which he sensed was growing among the rank and file. "There is a sign of [God's] visitation in the confrontation with the whole conscience factor as we are moving into our society.... I have moved among the folks now called Baptists for about twenty years, urging everybody to get involved, but I said when I want to get involved, I want to get involved with my understanding of values. And now they are all marching down to get involved and take charge of things, and I'm getting nervous about that."[2]

Many of the changes which Allen presaged have indeed come to pass, at least within the denomination over which he presided as the last moderate president. At the 1982 SBC in New Orleans, the substance of the 1980 resolution on abortion was expanded to declare "all human life, both born and pre-born, is sacred, bearing the image of God, and is not subject to personal judgments as to 'quality of life' based on such subjective criteria as stage of development, abnormality, intelligence level, degree of dependency, cost of medical treatment, or inconvenience to parents."[3] This resolution also criticized infanticide, child abuse, and active euthanasia. Two years later in Kansas City, the Convention went beyond a stance of negative opposition to abortion to encouraging Southern Baptists "to provide counseling, housing, and adoption placement services for unwed mothers."[4] Three years later, in 1987, the Christian Life Commission sponsored its first national conference on abortion. The theme was "Choosing Life: Southern Baptists and Abortion." At the same time, the Home Mission Board began to train churches for ministry in crisis pregnancy centers. In January 1988, the Sanctity of Human Life Sunday was placed on the denominational calendar for the first time (against, it might be said, the entrenched opposition of the former leaders of the CLC).

This shift has produced a new alignment between denominational programs and the Southern Baptist constituency. At the same time, Southern Baptists have also reached out in partnership with other evangelical groups on issues of life and death. This new alliance has produced quizzical looks on the part of many veterans of the moral and cultural wars that rage in our society. As Fred Loper, a family practice doctor, has expressed it: "Southern Baptists...have been conspicuous until the last few years only by their relative absence from the field. That makes us stand out. There are other people in the field, at least. We may not necessarily like what they do, but they are at least out there. That is the criticism of us: 'Where have you been?'"[5] As a matter of fact, Southern Baptists were not completely absent from the abortion conflict prior to the eighties. Individual Southern Baptists served on groups such as the Christian Action Council and the National Right to Life Committee. In addition, Baptists for Life, chaired by Bob Holbrook, a Baptist pastor in Texas, circulated literature and sought to raise the consciousness of Southern Baptists on issues of life and death.

All the same, in an historical survey of Catholic and Baptist positions on abortion done in 1975, McLeod Bryan could find no prominent Baptist ethicist who had contributed significantly or written extensively on behalf of the pro-life position. Bryan's study was part of a ground-breaking dialogue between Catholics and Baptists on abortion, a seminar jointly sponsored by the U.S. Conference of Catholic Bishops and the Ecumenical Institute of Wake Forest University in November, 1975. Bryan began his study by asserting that opposition to abortion was a common position shared historically by these two diverse Christian traditions. "We could almost present the historical positions of Catholics and Baptists in a single sentence," he said. "Abortion is murder and altogether forbidden at any stage and under any circumstance—a position endorsed historically by both Catholics and Baptists." However, Bryan went on to show how this consensus, which he perhaps overstated a bit too starkly, had already begun to break down by the mid 1970s.[6]

On the one hand, he noted a growing ferment among Catholic moral theologians toward a more laxist, contextual approach to issues of sexual ethics, including homosexuality and abortion. Among the advocates of this growing plurality of methodology and a more permissive stance on abortion were scholars such as Charles Curran, Daniel Maguire, Thomas O'Donnell, Daniel Callahan, and the feminist theologian Mary Daly. From various perspectives all of these writers were challenging the historic Catholic consensus against abortion and the magisterial authority of the church which had promulgated it.

On the Baptist side, of course, there was no such comparable body of highly developed tradition nor a superimposing magisterial hierarchy to undergird it. For this very reason, the slippage of Baptist leaders away from the historic consensus Bryan noted was accomplished much more easily and with less public fanfare. Thus Baptist leaders were among the early supporters of the Religious Coalition for Abortion Rights whose stated purpose was "to encourage and coordinate support for safe-guarding the legal option of abortion; for ensuring the right of individuals to make decisions in accordance with their consciences; and for opposing efforts to deny this right of conscience through constitutional amendment, or federal and state legislation."[7] Similarly, American Baptist pastor Howard Moody welcomed the *Roe v. Wade* decision in this way: "I am delighted. This is a landmark in relation to woman's rights."[8]

With other abortion-rights activists, Reverend Moody had pioneered a clergy abortion counseling service near his congregation.

Among Southern Baptists, this position was represented by Dr. Andrew Lester, who published an article on "The Abortion Dilemma" in the Baptist journal, *Review and Expositor,* in the spring of 1971. Although written two years before *Roe v. Wade,* this article utilized the same terminology of Justice Blackmun in referring to the unborn child as "potential human life." Arguing from a contextual ethical perspective, Lester asserted that whatever rights might be accorded to the conceptus were perforce overridden by the rights of "those human beings who are actualized— functioning in the world with responsibilities, developed talents, and active relationships—all of whom should be given higher value than the potential human life residing in the fertilized egg." Following this logic, he claimed that the decision to abort should include as valid considerations the physical and/or psychological health of the mother; the welfare of the family and/or society; and the kind of physical, psychological, and social existence the fetus would experience when born.[9]

Lest we think that the view presented in this article was an isolated opinion on the margins of SBC life, it is well to remember that in this same year—1971—the Southern Baptist Convention meeting in St. Louis passed its first resolution on abortion. While this resolution included a perfunctory tribute to the "sanctity of human life," it was in essence a strong call for the liberalizing and legalizing of abortion in this country. The resolution called for the legitimizing of abortion not only for the hard cases of rape, incest, fetal deformity, and threat to the life of the mother, but also "carefully ascertained evidence of the likelihood of damage to the emotional, mental, as well as physical health of the mother."[10] The language used in this resolution adopted by America's largest Protestant, and arguably most conservative, denomination was nearly identical to that of a similar resolution passed by the Unitarian-Universalist Association some eight years before.[11] Thus two years prior to the Supreme Court decision of 1973, which opened the floodgates to abortion on demand in the United States, the Southern Baptist Convention was on record advocating the decriminalization of abortion and extending the discretion of this decision into the realm of personal, privatized choice. The simple fact is that *Roe v. Wade* did little more than place a stamp of approval on what America's largest, most conservative Protestant denomination had already agreed to.

Lessons From History

The complicity and/or blindness of Southern Baptist leadership on such a critical moral front cannot be fully explained in terms of social, cultural, or church political trends. At the very heart of this ethical collapse was a profoundly theological failure of nerve. To illustrate this thesis, I want to refer to two episodes in the history of German Protestantism in the early twentieth century, both of which, I submit, form a gripping parallel to our own Southern Baptist situation on abortion.

The first incident involves the reaction of the Swiss pastor Karl Barth to the outbreak of the First World War on August 1, 1914. On that very day ninety-three German intellectuals issued a manifesto publicly identifying themselves with the war policy of Kaiser Wilhelm II, including the brutal violation of Belgian neutrality. At the time, Karl Barth was a minister in his first full-time church in the rural town of Safenwil in Switzerland. He was shocked to find among the signatories of the manifesto the names of almost all of his great German teachers, the theological masters with whom he had studied at Marburg and Berlin. From these great scholars he had imbibed the tradition of theological liberalism, which had hitherto guided his life and ministry as a pastor. "It was like the twilight of the gods," he said, "when I saw the reaction of Harnck, Hermann, Rade, Eucken and company to the new situation," and discovered how religion and scholarship could be changed completely "into intellectual 42 cm. canons."

The result was an experience of shattering disillusionment for the young Barth. "I did not know what to make of the teaching of all my theological masters in Germany. To me they seemed to be hopelessly compromised by what I regarded as their failure in the face of the ideology of war. Their 'ethical failure' indicated that their exegetical and dogmatic presuppositions could not be in order. Thus a whole world of exegeses, ethics, dogmatics and preaching, which I had hitherto held to be essentially trustworthy, was shaken to the foundations, and with it, all the other writings of the German theologians."[12] It was precisely this experience which prompted Barth to break with the liberal theology in which he had been trained so thoroughly and to begin to search for a new doctrinal orientation, a quest which led him to what he called "the strange new world within the Bible." While it may be true, as I believe, that Barth was never quite able to sever the umbilical cord which bound him to the very liberalism against which he protested, his realization that ethical outcome is directly related to theological foundation remains as true today as it was in 1914.

And what is true of individual believers, pastors, and theologians is also *a fortiori* true of the church as a corporate entity in its public witness. To move forward in German history from World War I to World War II, from Kaiser Wilheim II to Reichsfuhrer Adolf Hitler, is to raise the question of the resistance, or lack thereof, of the Christian churches in Germany to the Jewish policies of National Socialism. James Burtchaell, among others, has studied the record and motivation of the movement that affected the Holocaust with its eight million victims. They have discovered in the rhetoric and rationale of this movement a chilling analog to the movement advocating elective abortions in our own culture, a movement which can boast over 30 million victims in the past twenty years. For example, both movements are characterized by the depersonalization of the victims. The Jews in Nazi Germany were referred to as *Untermenschen,* subhumans. Other antisocials—the mentally ill, the physically deformed, the racially impure—were also denied the designation human [*Mensch*]. They were referred to by the German justice ministry as the *Missgeburten der Hîlle,* "the miscarriages of hell," fit only to be eliminated.[13] We are all too familiar with the euphemistic and derogatory nomenclature applied to the unborn in our own society today. The unborn have been designated as "protoplasmic rubbish," "a gobbet of meat protruding from a human womb," "the fetal-placental unit," "fallopian and uterine cell matter," "the products of pregnancy," "sub-human non-personhood," and so on.[14]

It is not our purpose to pursue this analogy further, but rather to point out the glaring silence and line of least resistance put forth by the major culture-shaping Christian traditions in the face of both holocausts. As Nazi anti-Semitism moved from theory to praxis, the Christian leaders of Germany were reluctant to speak against this state-sponsored, legally sanctioned policy of violence, although many of them feared the worst. While there were halting protests along the way, most of them were theologically ungrounded and politically ineffective. For example, the Nuremberg Laws were objected to not on the ground that all Jews were fellow human beings created in the image of God and thus entitled to a basic right to life, but rather on the self-serving and expedient grounds that certain Christian Jews would be swept along in a general persecution of all Jewish ethnics. As has been noted by others, "When the liquidation program moved East, turned genocidal, and swept away millions, it was then beyond the ability of the churches to oppose Hitler publicly and effectively. Nor did they try."[15]

The one major exception to this trend was the witness of the confessing church and its theology of resistance expressed in the Barmen Declaration of 1934. Here it was declared that the impregnable foundation of the Christian church is the gospel of Jesus Christ, revealed in Holy Scripture and reflected in the confessional heritage of the Reformation. As the signatories to the Barmen Declaration put it: "Precisely because we want to be and remain true to our various confessions of faith, we may not keep silent, for we believe that in a time of common need and trial (Anfechtung) a common word has been placed in our mouth."[16] The framers of Barmen rightly saw that the ethical nightmare which was about to seize the German people in 1934 was directly related to the dissolution of fundamental theological and confessional integrity among the churches. Here they took their stand, suffering the consequences of exile (Barth), imprisonment (Niemoeller), and death (Bonhoeffer).

Others chose to play it safe. Apart from Barmen, there was no concerted, public, official stand taken by any major Christian church in Germany against the Holocaust. Thus after the war the Protestant *Evangelische Kirche in Deutschland* confessed: "Before the God of mercy we share in the guilt for the outrage committed against the Jews by our own people through omission and silence."[17] The Baptist Union of Germany has recently issued a similar statement of contrition. Nor are Southern Baptists exempt from this incrimination. Many Southern Baptist leaders attended the Baptist World Alliance Congress in Berlin in 1936. They met under the banner of the swastika, received greetings from Hitler, and returned to America with glowing reports of the great things happening in Germany. They specifically minimized the totalitarianism and glaring anti-Semitism which was obvious even in 1936.[18]

A Loss of Vision

With these historical lessons in mind, I am ready now to state the central thesis: *The failure of the Southern Baptist Convention to make a timely and prophetic response to the holocaust of abortion on demand reflects the loss of theological vision resulting in the malign neglect and distorted understanding of the most basic doctrinal affirmations we profess to believe.* It is beyond the scope of this presentation to give an account of how this slippage came about. Elsewhere I have suggested that it is related to the loss of intentional Christian instruction and congregational discipline within our churches, together with a pervasive philosophy of pragmatism in church life which has produced quantitative success at the expense of theological identity.[19] Put otherwise, the problem is not merely that we have had a few theological liberals in our seminaries and denominational bureaucracy. That is the mere outcropping of a more basic and systemic problem; namely, the erosion of doctrinal substance and the failure to think through theologically the great issues of our time. Only this kind of slippage can account for the fact that the entire Convention in 1971 was willing to follow willy-nilly the directives of its denominational elites on an issue of such profound moral and social consequence.

If this line of reasoning is at all valid, it has important implications not only for the analysis of recent trends in SBC life, but also for the future directions we must take. I, for one, regard the reversal of the denominational trends of the sixties and seventies as a providential moving of God in our midst. Had we continued along the so-called progressivist trajectory we had set during those turbulent decades, we undoubtedly would have become just another mainline Protestant denomination, bereft of our missionary and evangelistic zeal and tossed and turned by every new-wave ideology which comes down the pike. For this rescue all of us who care deeply about the great heritage which has shaped our beloved denomination can give thanks to God. However, a word of warning is also in order: The mere replacement of one set of bureaucrats with another doth not a Reformation make. Unless there is genuine spiritual and theological renewal within our churches, the very pro-life views we have come lately to espouse could well be eroded under the pressures of an increasingly hostile political environment.

It is well to remember that the pro-life position gained wide acceptance across Southern Baptist life in the context of a political climate that was at least partially favorable to the protection of the unborn. We face the very real possibility of the passage of the Freedom of Choice Act, militant abortion-rights lobbying within every level of society, and the probability of a Supreme Court which will likely back further and further away from the *Webster* decision, with a reversal of *Roe v. Wade* becoming more and more remote in the foreseeable future. Unless our ethical positions are grounded in something more enduring than the shifting sands of Realpolitik, we may well pass on to the rising generation the same kind of vacuous mind-set which produced our denominational paralysis at the beginning of the pro-life struggle some thirty years ago. What is called for is a more thorough grounding of the ethics of life in the basic theological fundamentals of our evangelical Baptist and Christian heritage. The Christian Life Commission, together with the Sunday School Board and the Home Mission Board, have a special role to play as agencies charged by our Convention with developing resources and opportunities for ministry in this area. However, the theological renewal that must come cannot be a trickle-down phenomenon. It must arise from the conscientious commitment of every pastor, every Sunday School teacher, every student minister and Christian social worker, every professor in every seminary and college classroom across our beloved Convention. What we need is not only social awareness and political activism but theological revival!

Theological Roots

I want to turn now to examine briefly three major doctrinal loci, each of which is crucial for an ethic of life that is both grounded in the witness of Holy Scripture and faithful to the evangelical heritage of the Baptist tradition. We shall look briefly, then, at the doctrine of God, the Incarnation, and the mission of the church.

For the past decade and a half, theological controversy among Southern Baptists has focused almost exclusively on the authority and inspiration of the Bible. This issue became a matter of public concern because the total truthfulness of God's Word had been compromised in certain quarters by blatant concession to a destructive form of historical-critical methodology. On numerous occasions since 1963, when the Baptist Faith and Message was adopted, Southern Baptists have affirmed an unswerving commitment to the divine inspiration and inerrancy of Holy Scripture, the Word of God revealed in written form. Those Southern Baptists who have argued for the moral acceptability of abortion have chosen not to challenge this basic Baptist commitment. Rather, they have argued that their own position is really more, not less, biblical than that of their pro-life opponents, citing the fact that the Bible nowhere specifically says, "Thou shalt not have an abortion." Of course, it is also true that the Bible nowhere says thou shalt not commit uxoricide, the murder of one's wife, nor infanticide, the murder of a post-born child. However, behind the hermeneutical squabble over biblical evidence for or against abortion looms a larger, often unnoticed, theological premise; namely, the nature and character of the very God who inspired the Bible in the first place.

The doctrine of God is the cornerstone of Christian theology. Historically, Baptists have affirmed, along with other believers in the classical Christian tradition, the sovereignty and aseity of the one eternal God of Holy Scripture who both knows Himself and has made Himself known to us as Father, Son, and Holy Spirit. We confess that God is infinite in all perfections, which means that He is all-sufficient, neither standing in need of any creatures He has made, nor deriving any glory from them, but rather manifesting His own glory in, by, unto, and upon them. This God is the fountain of all being. He alone is the inexhaustible source of all life, glory, goodness, and blessedness. He is all-knowing, all-powerful, and omnipresent. God is utterly transcendent, graciously beneficent, and immutably just in all His dealing with humankind.

It is precisely this God, and not another, who has created human beings, males and females, in His own image, only in virtue of which do they possess "the right to life." An ethic of life encompasses both the doctrines of creation and providence. Human beings derive their origin by a direct act of God initiated in the divine counsel ("Let us make man in our own image..."). The *imago dei* signifies that every human being stands in a direct and inviolable relation to the Creator. What is important to recognize here is that in creating human life and endowing it with His own divine image, God was moved by no necessity nor constraint either internal or external to His own being, but solely by what the New Testament calls the *eudokia,* the good pleasure, of His divine will. This means quite simply that at the most basic level human beings are not necessary in an ontological or metaphysical sense. God would have been not one whit less God had He chosen not to create the world or human beings within it.

However, rather than mitigating the significance of human life, this truth underscores its abiding validity and unique importance. Since God has chosen to invest His own glory in creatures made in His own image, then the inviolability and independent integrity of that life must be protected even, nay especially, in its embryonic development. The assault upon the unborn is nothing less than an attack upon the Creator of life itself.

An example of the theological confusion related to this very basic point is seen in David Hughes' claim that we should ditch the term "sanctity of human life" in favor of the more general "respect" or "reverence for life."[20] This latter term, of course, is associated with Albert Schweitzer, the great philanthropist and liberal theologian, whose radical biblical scholarship led him to abandon every vestige of orthodox, supernaturalist Christianity in favor of a kind of pantheistic spirituality. While we may all applaud Schweitzer's sacrificial exploits as a missionary doctor in Africa, we dare not follow his rejection of the central biblical and

Christological affirmations of the Christian faith. The word *sanctus* means not only "holy" but also "set apart." In the biblical perspective, human life is both holy and set apart from all other forms of finite life by virtue of its capacity to bear the image of the Triune God.

Certainly we must reject the kind of myopic logic that sees obligations to life *in utero* but fails to accept responsibility for the quality of life *extra uterum*. However, it is the sanctity of human life and not a mere reverence for life in general that underscores the integrity and eternal value of the *humanum* from inception to death, a death which we cannot believe the gracious God intended to occur by violent human intrusion even prior to birth. Thus, the sanctity of human life extends back to one's beginnings, deriving as it does from the holy and set-apart God, maker of heaven and earth, in whom we live, move, and have our being.

It is significant that Southern Baptist advocates of pro-choice have themselves identified the doctrine of God as the crucial theological divide on the issue of abortion. For example, Paul Simmons has written:

> One of the most glaring weaknesses in the fundamentalist theology regarding abortion is its doctrine of providence. What is at issue is the way in which God is related to the entire process of conception and birth or the processes of nature as such. For fundamentalists, God is the cause and power of all that is; God governs all natural processes. This is important for them in supporting the absolutism of their stance against abortion....What is at stake in the fundamentalist's posture is a Calvinistic stress on the sovereignty of God.[21]

Dr. Simmons then proceeds to identify three profound theological problems caused by this skewed view of God's providence: (1) The goodness of God is compromised in favor of God's power. This turns God into a cruel deity and prompts fundamentalists to reject "scientific notions of chance and randomness that work in the creative process and thus react strongly to any notion that God is not totally in control." (2) Human beings are seen as passive victims who can only bear whatever tragedy may befall. "It is unthinkable to argue that people, made in the image of God, may have to make some god-like decisions regarding our stewardship of procreative powers, as in abortion." (3) A limited and inadequate view of grace does not give permission "to act with boldness in spite of ambiguity."[22] Taken together these arguments clearly show how the abandonment of the historic Baptist doctrine of God and His providence made possible the justification and acceptance of a pro-choice ideology among various leaders within the Southern Baptist Convention.

The biblical doctrine of providence, affirmed by historic Baptist confessions, refers to God's daily care for all creatures, His divine guidance of the course of human history, and indeed His infallible ordering of the entire cosmos so as to accomplish what He has purposed for all eternity to do. Put otherwise, God's providential activity encompasses His *preservation* of creation, His *direction* of all things toward their ultimate goal, and His *governance* of every event, circumstance, and process toward the consummation of all things which will be accomplished in God's own time. God's sovereignty and providence do not entail fatalism, since God works in such a way that human free will is sustained and human responsibility is required. On the other hand, the pro-choice theology of providence seems to involve a mixture of deism and chance. God appears as the *deus otiosus,* the lazy god who observes human events from a far distance, leaving the world He has made to run its course more or less on its own. Within this world randomness or chance is at work wreaking havoc throughout the created realm.

Over against this view, Baptists have historically confessed, with orthodox Christians everywhere, that the God we worship and serve is the omnipotent Lord of time and eternity. There is no random force, no gaping chaos, no spiritual black hole, over which He is not the supreme Lord and ultimate victor. This view of God's providence does not solve all the hard cases related to abortion. But it does provide a theological foundation for affirming God's sustaining presence and overcoming grace in every tragic situation which occurs in our fallen world. In the face of suffering and tragedy and questions which submit to no easy answers, true piety will realize that behind the hurt we experience, God remains in His justice, wisdom, and love the Father who has promised never to leave or forsake us. Far from inspiring passive resignation or bitter outrage, this doctrine of providence has sustained countless men and women in moments of crisis, danger, and death.

While historic Baptist theology affirms without compromise the sovereignty and providential governance of Almighty God, this God is not to be equated with the First Cause, Unmoved Mover, or Final Force of Aristotelian metaphysics. At the heart of the Christian message, indeed that which characterizes it as gospel, good news, is the proclamation that this omnipotent, eternal God has chosen not to spend eternity with Himself, "the alone with the alone," as Arius put it. The God of creation is also the Lord of redemption. In the person of His Son Jesus Christ God has intimately identified Himself with the human condition, as a baby in a manger, as a man on a cross. It is part of the offense of particularity that when God became man, He did not bypass our humanity but came into the very thick of it with genes and chromosomes and a fingerprint of His own.

Advocates of elective abortion, including some Southern Baptists, have seized upon the fact that the New Testament nowhere explicitly condemns this practice. As one of them has recently put it: "The biblical writer's silence on abortions reveals a reticence to judge too quickly concerning the morality of another person's choice. It is eloquent testimony to the sacredness of this choice for women and their families and the privacy in which it is to be considered."[23] Indeed, we are tempted to think that we would be spared many useless debates had the Holy Spirit seen fit to inspire one of the biblical writers to include a prohibition of abortion among one of the various lists of sinful vices in the ancient world. We should be careful, however, in jumping too hastily to this conclusion since the repeated condemnation of homosexual behavior in the New Testament has done little to prevent certain Christians, including some Southern Baptists, from ignoring and circumventing its plain meaning.

On the other hand, Michael J. Gorman, among others, has argued that the silence of the New Testament on this issue, far from implying neutrality or ambiguity, simply reflected the continuation of the pro-life norm inherited from Judaism.[24] Moreover, when the abortion temptation did arise as a specific problem, the church answered with an unequivocal no. This is clearly borne out in early Christian writings such as the *Didache,* the Epistle of Barnabas, the Apocalypse of Peter, not to mention the more explicit condemnations of later church fathers such as Minucius Felix, Tertullian, Cyprian, Chrysostom, Jerome, Augustine, and others. That the anti-abortion stance of the early church was a matter of public witness, and not merely private belief, is borne out by the statement of Athenagoras, a second-century apologist, who addressed this statement to the emperor, Marcus Aurelius: "How can we kill a man when we are those who say that all who use abortifacients are homicides and will account to God for their abortions as for the killing of men? For the fetus in the womb is not an animal, and it is God's providence that he exists."[25]

Other scholars have pointed to various strands in the literature of the New Testament which, when taken together, certainly anticipate the explicit consensus of the early church teaching on the sanctity of human life. For example, when Joseph discovered the unexpected pregnancy of his teenage fiancee, he contemplated divorce but not abortion. We see Jesus' concern and identification with the "least of these," including the vulnerable, the helpless, "the little ones," offense against whom He warned would surely bring divine judgment; the listing of *pharmakeia* in Gal. 5:19-21, arguably a warning against the use of abortion-inducing drugs; the love commandment and the Golden Rule together with the extraordinary interest in the fetal and infant life of Jesus himself as reflected in the infancy narratives.[26]

While all of these texts have important implications for a contemporary ethic of life, to my mind the central New Testament text on this issue is John 1:14: "And the Word was made flesh and dwelt among us, (and we beheld his glory, the glory of the only begotten of the Father,) full of grace and truth." This verse has tremendous implications for Christian anthropology for, as John Calvin wisely noted, the full meaning of the image of God can be nowhere better recognized than in the restoration of our corrupted nature in the incarnate Son of God, the second Adam, in whom alone our true and complete humanity is restored. (Institutes 1.15.4).

Fundamental to the reality of the Incarnation is the unity of body and soul, as distinct from various kinds of Greek and Eastern dualism. The eternal word, *Logos,* could not have become flesh, *sarx,* if this unity were not the distinctive reality of human beings. The God-man is at once the true pattern of authentic human personhood and the divine word of life itself.

The Johannine text asserts what to the Greek mind was unthinkable, *ho logos egeneto sarx*, "the Word became flesh." It does not say that the Word merely assumed a human person. That would have been conceivable and more palatable to the Greek mind, as the gods of Olympus often masqueraded as human characters. However, to assert so boldly that the Word became flesh is to claim that God Himself has entered the human arena at its most vulnerable point. So central was this affirmation to the New Testament church that Christians are admonished to regard as antichrist anyone who denies that Jesus Christ has come in the flesh (1 John 4:2-3).

Over against the doctrine of the Incarnation stands the docetic Christology of gnosticism with its disparagement of matter. In this view the body is beyond redemption; the true self is the spirit or soul within. We are witnessing the revival of gnostic anthropology in the modern movement for elective abortions. One advocate of this position has claimed: "Humans are actual spirits. The spirit exists prior to birth and will go on existing after the body dies. I propose that the spirit of a particular human enters the body along with the first breath of air. Not until the first voluntary breath of the child is the full-fledged human present."[27] In the face of the gnostic disparagement of human reality, the early church pointed to the centrality of the Incarnation, confessing that Jesus Christ was truly (*althos*) conceived in the womb of the Virgin Mary by the power of the Holy Spirit; He was truly born in the manger of Bethlehem, He truly lived, truly died on the cross, and truly rose from the grave. In like manner, He will truly come again and thus we confess our faith in the resurrection of the body, not just the reabsorption of the spirit into the divine promira. In the face of contemporary theories of human development which marginalize the sacred value of unborn human life, we can do no better than to echo the words of the apostle Paul, "When the time had fully come, God sent His Son, born of a woman" (Gal. 4:4, NIV).

The Christological consensus which sustained the confessing church in Nazi Germany must undergird our own efforts to bear a faithful witness in the midst of our *Kirchenkampf* today. In solidarity with Barmen, we too confess:

> Jesus Christ, as he has testified to us in the Holy
> Scripture, is the one Word of God, whom we are to hear,
> whom we are to trust and obey in life and in death....
> Just as Jesus Christ is the pledge of the forgiveness of
> all our sins, just so—and with the same earnestness—
> He is also God's mighty claim on the entirety of human
> life; in Him we encounter a joyous liberation from the
> godless claims of this world to free and thankful service
> to His creatures.[28]

The erosion of theological and Christological foundations in our common life as Southern Baptists has also called into question our identity and mission as a corporate people of God called to bear witness in a culture of decline. Again and again, Southern Baptist advocates for abortion rights have appealed to traditional Baptist notions of soul competency, religious liberty, and the priesthood of all believers as a rationale for relegating the decision to abort to the realm of privatized morality. For example, in an article published by Americans United for the Separation of Church and State, it is boldly stated that abortion should be legally available to every woman, "the moral agents whose rights are uniquely at stake. Gestating life should be seen in terms of its value to the woman, the couple or society itself, and not in terms of obvious or intrinsic personhood."[29] Still another Baptist ethicist has written, "Our Baptist heritage is clear on this matter. We must stand for the liberty to choose: whether to bear a child or withdraw life support from a fetus.... The freedom of the individual to choose is paramount and must not be sacrificed to rhetoric that deifies the conceptus making personal freedom subject to biological determinism."[30]

Baptists do indeed have a splendid history as champions of religious liberty, a record from which we dare not retreat, especially in a time and nation where this precious freedom is increasingly under attack. The Baptist commitment to religious liberty, however, has never been a pretext either for doctrinal indifference or moral laxity. The doctrine of religious liberty claims the right of every congregation to order its own internal life, its doctrine and discipline, in accordance with its own perception of divine truth. It requires that there be no external political monitoring of the internal religious life of voluntary associations. However, historically this principle has never meant, and it must not now be twisted to mean, that Baptists must wink at theological heresy in the name of tolerable diversity, or that they must be silent in the face of outrageous moral evil within the environing culture which surrounds them.

As I have argued elsewhere, the priesthood of all believers has more to do with the Christian's service than with his status.[31] It is not a prerogative on which we can rest; it is a commission which sends us forth into the world to exercise a priestly ministry not for ourselves, but for others—the outsiders—not instead of Christ, but for the sake of Christ and at His behest. To reduce the decision of abortion to the level of privatized morality is to equate Christianity with a kind of modern individualism which in its flight from community and responsibility is the very antithesis of the biblical metaphor of the church as the body of Christ, a pilgrim people bound together in covenant one with another and with God, a prophetic company of called-out ones charged by Christ Himself to shine forth as lights and to season as salt in a world which has lost its moral bearings. There is, of course, another side to this kind of costly witness: the call not only to be against promiscuous abortions, but also the mandate to stand beside those caught up in the trauma of such an act, the proclamation of forgiveness, the extension of compassion, the love of Christ which reaches out to embrace, to restore, and to heal. If all we have to offer is a raucous protest to the evil about us, then we have not yet come to truly know our Savior in the *koinonia* of His sufferings and the power of His resurrection.

It is ironic, perhaps, that the church of Jesus Christ finds itself today in a position quite similar to one which prevailed at the beginning of the Christian era. In those days it was surrounded by a society in which abortion and infanticide were practiced frequently. Drawing on the biblical and theological substance of the Christian faith, it stood over against the culture and combated this evil in word and deed. As my own professor and mentor, George Hunston Williams of Harvard has pointed out, it is anomalous that at the very moment when we know the most about the process of conception and prenatal life, we are witnessing the devolution of the moral conscience of society back toward a pagan, pre-Christian disregard for the sanctity of human life, a retreat led in many quarters by the very professions, medical, legal, and yes religious, which should be pledged to its protection.[32]

If Southern Baptists are to maintain a consistent Christian witness on issues of life and death in this kind of increasingly hostile environment, then we must dig down to the deep roots and firm foundations of the faith that was once for all entrusted to the saints, to the end that we be no longer children, tossed by the waves and whirled about by every fresh gust of teaching, duped by crafty rogues and their deceitful schemes. Rather, we must speak the truth in love, and thus shall we fully grow up into Christ. May God help us so to live and so to act and so to speak.

Endnotes

[1]*Ethical Issues for the Eighties.* 1980 Christian Life Commission Seminar Proceedings.

[2]Ibid., 59. See Timothy George, "Toward an Evangelical Future," *Southern Baptists Observed: Multiple Perspectives on a Changing Denomination*, ed. Nancy Tatom Ammerman (Knoxville: University of Tennessee Press, 1993), 276-300.

[3]Annual of the Southern Baptist Convention, 1982, 65.

[4]Annual of the Southern Baptist Convention, 1984, 66.

[5]*Choosing Life: Southern Baptists and Abortion.* Proceedings of the 1987 National Conference on Abortion, 11.

[6]*Seminar on Abortion.* Proceedings of a Dialogue Between Catholics and Baptists (November 10-12, 1975), 10. In the 1940s theology professor Harold W. Tribble openly referred to abortion as murder in his classes at Southern Seminary. Personal conversation with Fred M. Wood, May 27, 1993.

[7]"A Call to Concern," Religious Coalition for Abortion Rights.

[8]*Seminar on Abortion*, 17.

[9]Andrew Lester, "The Abortion Dilemma,"*Review and Expositor* 67 (1971), 233.

[10]Annual of the Southern Baptist Convention, 1971, 72.

[11]George Huntston Williams, "Religious Residues and Presuppositions in the American Debate on Abortion," *Theological Studies* 31 (1970), 51.

[12]Eberhard Busch, *Karl Barth* (Philadelphia: Fortress Press, 1976), 81 .

[13]James T. Burtchaell, *Rachel Weeping: The Case Against Abortion* (San Francisco: Harper and Row, 1978), 148.

[14]Ibid., 196.

[15]Ibid., 183.

[16]*Creeds of the Churches*, ed. John H. Leith (Atlanta: John Knox Press, 1982), 519.

[17]Burtchaell, *Rachel Weeping*, 183.

[18]Cf. William Loyd Allen, "How Baptists Assessed Hitler," *The Christian Century,* (Sept. 1, 1982), 891-92.

[19]Timothy George, "Conflict and Identity in the SBC: The Quest for a New Consensus," *Beyond the Impasse?: Scripture, Interpretation, and Theology in Baptist Life*, eds. Robison B. James and David S. Dockery (Nashville: Broadman Press, 1992), 195-214.

[20]David Hughes, "Paying Our Respects to Life," *Global Discipleship*. Published by the Cooperative Baptist Fellowship.

[21]Paul D. Simmons, "A Theological Response to Fundamentalism on the Abortion Issue," in *Abortion: The Moral Issues,* Edward Batchelor, Jr. (New York: Pilgrim Press, 1982), 180.

[22]Ibid., 180-182.

[23]Paul D. Simmons, *Personhood, the Bible, and the Abortion Debate*, quoted in Michael J. Gorman, "Why Is the New Testament Silent About Abortion?" *Christianity Today,* (January 11, 1993), 28.

[24]Ibid.

[25]Athenagoras, *Patrologia Graeca* 6.919.

[26]See John T. Noonan, "An Almost Absolute Value in History," in *The Morality of Abortion*, ed. John T. Noonan (Cambridge, Mass.: Harvard University Press, 1970), 1-59.

[27]Warren F. Metzler, "Why Abortion Isn't Murder," *First Things* 31 (March, 1993), 4.

[28]*Creeds of the Churches*, 520-521.

[29]Paul D. Simmons, "Dogma and Discord: Religious Liberty and the Abortion Debate," *Church and State* (January, 1990), 18.

[30]Howard Moody, "Baptists and Freedom: Some Reminders and Remembrances of Our Past for the Sake of Our Present," *American Baptist Quarterly* vol. 3 (March 1984) 8-9.

[31]Timothy George, "The Priesthood of All Believers and the Quest for Theological Integrity," *Criswell Theological Review* 3 (1989), 283294. For a discussion of how the "right to life" has been overridden by the "right to privacy," see Larry R. Churchill and Jose Jorge Siman, "Abortion and the Rhetoric of Individual Rights," *Hastings Center Report* 12 (1982), 9-12.

[32]George Huntston Williams, "The Sacred Condominium," in *The Morality of Abortion*, 171.

PART II
Human Genetics

The Human Genome Project

By Francis Collins

I do not carry any special credentials in the field of ethics, but I think there are certain aspects of medicine that I understand pretty well, and which I believe carry an enormous number of challenges for the future. I believe the church needs to be prepared for these challenges.

I have on my wall a hanging which my daughter did for me in calligraphy. It is based on a quote from James 1:5, NASB, "If any man lacks wisdom, let him ask of God, who gives to all men generously and without reproach, and it will be given to him." This points, of course, to the source of all genuine wisdom. I pray that more of the world would appreciate this fact.

My favorite quote from Winston Churchill is that "Success is nothing more than going from failure to failure with undiminished enthusiasm." This is worth remembering. In many endeavors of life, where your first try or your second or your ninety-fourth does not seem to quite do it, perhaps the ninety-fifth will. Certainly the challenges that face Christians today could be couched in those terms. Yet we must remember that we have right on our side.

I grew up in a fairly high-church Episcopal background. I learned a lot about music and not a thing about theology. When I got to college, as many do, I found my faith challenged by those around me who did not have much use for it. I discovered that I did not know enough about my faith to be able to defend it, so it quickly slipped away from me. I skidded back into agnosticism and eventually into atheism, where I stayed fairly comfortably for a period of about ten years. Then I began to feel vaguely, and later profoundly, uneasy about my failure to have ever really considered the evidence for what is clearly the most important question of life; that is, is there a God, and did He have a Son named Jesus Christ who came to earth and died on a cross?

After a lot of running away from that question, I was introduced to the writings of C. S. Lewis, which were perfect for me. They torpedoed all of the convenient arguments I had put together about the irrationality of faith and replaced them with arguments about the irrationality of unbelief, which certainly is a more powerful set of arguments when you compare them. And so, at the age of twenty-seven, I had a genuine conversion experience and became a Christian in a serious sort of way. For the last seven years I have been a Southern Baptist, and that has been a wonderful source of guidance, warmth, comfort, fellowship, and belief for me.

Often in my career as a physician-geneticist I feel as though I am on a mission field because science and Christianity seem to be at loggerheads. In my view this is unfortunate. We are facing a series of advances in genetic medicine that are going to have awesome consequences. I believe those advances have great potential to alleviate suffering and save lives, but I also believe they have some potential for misuse. The church must get involved in a constructive way in discussing that potential. I suspect these issues are going to move along more quickly than some of us would like.

Science and the church do not have a pretty history. Yet, as both a scientist and a Christian, I see no discordance at all between what I believe as a Christian and what science teaches me about the world. In fact, I would venture to say that, for the scientist who is also a Christian, science is a form of worship. It is an uncovering of the incredible, awesome beauty of God's creation. That is how I feel when I have a chance to glimpse something which no human being previously knew—but God knew all along. I do not think any true believer should really fear science. Is science going to disprove faith? Surely not. The real issue is, to what extent will the knowledge that science produces become used in a way that is damaging to what we all hold dear? The *use* of information is certainly something in which the church ought to be involved.

Since the Genome Project is still a very unfamiliar series of terms and jargon, let me describe just a little bit of the basic background. First, I direct you to a proverb which is ignored at their peril by both scientists and Christians: "It is not good to have zeal without knowledge." The church is therefore obligated to acquire knowledge in areas that require thorny ethical decisions to be made. It is not sufficient to take a stand against something without understanding what that something is. Scientists obviously have knowledge in certain areas and severely lack it in others; sometimes their zeal gets a little out of hand as well.

If you are passing newsstands these days, you certainly are assaulted with information about genetics. Some of it is real, some a bit overblown. *U.S. News and World Report, Time,* and even *Consumer Reports* have carried cover stories on genes and heredity. But what is "DNA" anyway? It is the blueprint, the chemical inside the nucleus of the cell, that carries the instructions that allow that cell (and the whole organism, the human body) to carry out the series of steps that we all have to do in order to maintain ourselves against a barrage of outside influences. It also puts organs together and all those things that a cell has to do in order to move from that one-celled embryo into a fully formed organism. DNA, however, as the blueprint, is not itself very active biochemically. The way it does its job is to be copied into RNA, and then that RNA is translated into protein, which really does the job.

So how does a genetic disease occur? It occurs if there is an alteration in the DNA, which then results in an abnormality in the RNA, which then leads to a protein problem. The consequence of the disease comes about because the protein is not working, but the basic defect is in the DNA. If you really want to understand a genetic disease, you need to understand it at the DNA level.

DNA is actually a rather simple structure. It is made up of a wonderful double helix, and at each position along that double helix there is one of four possible so-called bases. Every possibility is either A, C, G, or T. If you have an A on one strand, you pair with a T on the other, and C always pairs with G, so if you know one strand you automatically know the other. The blueprint can be thought of as a series of encyclopedias written in this special four-letter language, where each word is made up of a series of As, Cs, Gs, and Ts. That information content is what allows the organism to do all the things it has to do.

The DNA is not just thrown into the nucleus of the cell in totally random, tangled fashion. It is wound up into chromosomes, which you can actually see under a microscope. These come in pairs—twenty-two of them—one from your father and one from your mother going into each pair. Each one of those chromosomes has a lot of genes on it. A gene is a stretch of DNA that codes for a particular protein. Genes vary in length, from short ones that may be only a few thousand base pairs to enormous ones that are a couple of million base pairs. The unit length of DNA is a base pair, that is, the two strands of DNA paired together. On a given chromosome there are thousands of genes. In fact, the total number of genes in man is about one hundred thousand, we think.

The whole thing—all of the DNA, all of the chromosomes, all of the genes—is called the genome, which is a word that people are really troubled about. It recently came into existence and was probably a poor choice for a project of such importance to have attached to it. Most people are immediately lost when you say, "Do you know something about the Genome Project?" They sort of scan their memory, trying to remember, "What is a genome?" It is just all of the above—all of that blueprint information.

These various genes can go awry. A catalog put out at Johns Hopkins seeks to keep track of all the inherited disorders of mankind that have been reported in the medical literature, but new ones are constantly being identified. At this point we know of about five thousand conditions that are presumably due to the action of one or more altered genes wreaking some havoc on the normal function of the body. For most of those diseases, we don't have a clue what the basic problem is. We can only catalog the conditions and scratch our heads. As recently as ten or twelve years ago, people would have said that most of those diseases are going to be totally unapproachable for the next century. You can describe them, you can talk about their natural history, but as far as really understanding them or treating them, it is pretty hopeless. The genome is too big; there are too many genes; you will never understand them all.

What has happened over the course of the last ten years is a remarkable acceleration in our ability to understand how genes work and to identify specific genes that cause specific diseases. We now have a paradigm that is followed when a disease needs to be figured out. I would argue strongly that if you want to understand a disease, you must understand it at its most basic level, which is the genetic alterations. Then you have the possibility of understanding it well enough to do something about it in the way of a treatment. When the gene is found, one often can identify abnormalities or mutations in that gene that occur in people with that disease. That gives you very quickly the ability to make diagnoses. It often takes much longer, however, from the time you found the gene, to develop enough information about that and understand it well enough to come up with a new treatment, be it a gene therapy or a drug therapy, and longer still to come to a cure.

The major dilemma we are about to face is the discovery of a whole host of genetic causes of disease, which puts us in the position of being able to be very good at diagnosing things. But time will need to pass, research will need to be done intensively before we will get to the point of being able to treat and cure those diseases. We are going to be faced with a window where our ability to understand and diagnose has gone far ahead of our ability to treat and cure. There is nothing we can do about that. You cannot get to treatment and cure without understanding the genetic basis of the disease. And understanding the genetic basis of the disease almost automatically tells you how to diagnose it. We will be caught in this situation for several decades with a large number of diseases.

What is so novel about the current research? Why did people say ten or twelve years ago that nobody could understand diseases of this sort? It is basically a problem of scale. The human genome is very large. It consists of about three billion base pairs. If you want to understand a disease, you may be looking for an abnormality that is as subtle as one single base pair that is not working out of that total of three billion. Sickle-cell anemia, for example, is a common, very severe genetic disease, primarily affecting individuals with an African background. One in five hundred blacks suffers from sickle-cell anemia. The disease affects multiple organ systems and leads to great suffering and premature death in many of those affected. That is all due to one residue on chromosome eleven that, instead of being an A is a T. One base pair out of three billion, if it is in the wrong place, is all it takes to give you sickle-cell anemia. And that will be true of many genetic diseases. That is why people would have said, "This is just too hard to solve," especially if you do not know anything ahead of time about most of these diseases, so you do not even know where to look.

If you are a little numbed by the idea of three billion base pairs, let me give you an analogy to try to show why this is a fairly remarkable achievement, even though it is now becoming almost routine. You are taking a photograph of someone having a picnic in a city park, but you take the picture from a satellite many miles out in space. If you are high enough, the person in the park may occupy one billionth of the field of the photograph. This is similar in scale to trying to spot the sickle-cell mutation in the midst of all those chromosomes.

Or, if you are trying to understand cystic fibrosis, which we knew almost nothing about until some four years ago, the situation is similar. In this case there are three base pairs involved. If you had to find the person in the photograph, how would you go about it? You probably would come up with some searching scheme that allowed you to narrow down the interval that you had to study, until gradually you got closer and closer and finally located the person. Every time you read about or hear on the news a description of the gene that causes Lou Gehrig's disease, for example, you can know that researchers have gone from outer space to the person in the park. They have done it again!

One reason these advances have become possible is the blossoming of this new idea—the Human Genome project—which is to build maps and determine basically the infrastructure of the human genome, to deduce the normal maps and sequences of large regions and eventually the whole thing, once and for all, in an organized way. This is the largest biomedical science endeavor ever undertaken. It is actually much less expensive, it turns out, than the supercollider or the space station, but for biology this is big science. This project, which has only officially been under way now for about two and a half years, currently has a budget of about one hundred million dollars per year. Some of that comes through the Department of Energy, but most of it comes through the National Institutes of Health. The project is targeted to take fifteen years, at the end of which, in the year 2005, all of the sequence—all of those As, Cs, Gs, and Ts—for the human genome will have been determined. That sequence will fill the equivalent of twenty-three sets of *Encyclopedia Britannica*. And the next several hundred years will be spent analyzing it and trying to figure out how it all works, because that will not be immediately obvious. All of those hundred thousand genes, however, will be identified in the process of determining those maps and sequences, so there will be an enormous amount of information that comes out of this project. And the ability to identify the genetic basis of disease will rapidly expand.

When I refer to genetic diseases, I am talking about cystic fibrosis and sickle-cell anemia, but I also am referring to problems that may be in your family. If you look carefully, there are almost no medical conditions that are not genetic. Perhaps trauma is an exception, but otherwise, even infectious diseases have a genetic connection. There is a reason why some people get various infectious diseases and other people do not, and that relates to their genetic make-up. Most people can think of some condition that runs in their family. All of us carry around somewhere between five and ten genes that have significant problems that are likely, at some point, to rear their heads and cause us to become ill. We are facing the possibility of being able to identify those in the course of the next ten to fifteen years. Are we ready for that? Are we ready for the consequences of that? Many of the consequences are going to be very good; some of the consequences are troublesome, and we must not shy away from them.

What the Genome Project is going to do is to figure out the whole sequence of all those chromosomes, once and for all. It will be done. This is a moment in history. It will only be done once. Other projects which have much more of the public's eye—space exploration, the supercollider, which will look at the structure of the nucleus—while having enormous appeal and enormous importance, pale by comparison to what we will learn about ourselves from the Genome Project. Alexander Pope said, "The proper study of man is man." And the Genome Project is studying man in a way never before possible.

As a result of this technology, some things have happened which are already spurring debates about the proper application of this information to the general public. Cystic fibrosis (CF) is the most common, potentially fatal disease of the Caucasian population. Most people know a child or have a family member with cystic fibrosis. It is dominated by lung problems—lungs that fill up with thick, sticky mucus that blocks air flow, leading to super infection with bacteria, and eventually causing the affected individual to suffocate. Much progress has been made using conservative symptomatic measures, so that the average individual with CF now lives to about age thirty, which is dramatically better than only twenty or thirty years ago. But the last few years of life are, in general, rather difficult, and it is not fair to say that we have adequate treatments for all stages of this disease. The hope for that lies in identifying the basic defect and then using that information to come up with a truly specific and effective therapy.

The inheritance of this disease is important. It is autosomal recessive, as many genetic diseases are, and that means an affected individual must have parents who *both* carry one abnormal copy of the gene and one normal one. The parents are healthy and have no inkling that they are carriers unless they happen to have a child to whom each of them passes along the altered gene and the child ends up affected. You have two copies of the CF genes. These are on chromosome seven. As long as one of them works you are okay. Only if both of them do not work will you have CF. The only way for that to happen is if both parents are carriers. In the past there was no way for individuals to know they were carriers for CF except by the experience of having an affected child. That has all changed. It is now possible to find out if you are a carrier for CF. Would you want to? That is the question that is being asked.

The gene was identified in 1989 by the very laborious process of coming in from outer space to the person in the park, ultimately identifying a subtle three base pair deletion that occurs in most individuals with CF, but not all. In fact, about 70 percent of CF alterations are due to this one change. The other 30 percent are due to a bunch of other changes in the same gene. If you want to detect all cases of cystic fibrosis, you have a tough time ahead of you. Those percentages vary in different parts of the world and with different ethnic groups. In the U.S., we can currently detect 85 percent of CF carriers by identifying a specific abnormality in the CF gene in those individuals, and we miss the other 15 percent because they have some other abnormality in the same gene that is harder to find. Eighty-five percent is still a lot of people.

One in twenty-five Caucasians is a carrier for CF. If they happen to be married to another individual who is a CF carrier, and they find this information out, they might choose not to have children, to adopt, or perhaps to go ahead and take their chances. Certainly there are couples out there who would like to have the chance to find out that information before proceeding with childbearing. So a debate has been raging in the genetics community and in the public health community about whether we should start offering, right now, CF carrier screening to the general population of the U.S. or even of the world. A few pilot projects have already gotten under way, and we all anxiously await the results.

What will people do with this information? Will they be glad to find this out, or will they wish they had never asked? What kinds of decisions will be made? Will people really understand what cystic fibrosis is? It is a very complicated disease that takes physicians years to learn about. How are you going to explain to a couple faced with the possibility of having a child with CF what the disease is? They are going to have to use that information to make an informed decision. It is a very hard problem. If you think that carrier screening is simple and that this could not possibly go awry, look back at the sickle-cell anemia carrier screening from the 1970s. A great deal of misinformation was passed along, and individuals who were carriers went away thinking they were going to develop sickle-cell anemia themselves. We cannot have another experience of that sort. I think the public would not forgive us, nor should they.

This issue is not yet resolved. The Office of Technology Assessment, an agency of the government, has recently come out with a report saying "The answer is 'Yes.' The only question is when." That is troubling to some of us, because I do not know that there is enough information to say that doing this is definitely a good idea.

Another question is, at what point will screening be carried out? As a Christian who believes in the sanctity of life and who believes in Psalm 139, I believe that individuals ought to have this information, if they are going to, in a way that allows them to take advantage of that before a pregnancy is already under way. My colleagues in the genetics community do not all agree with that. I regret to say that most CF carrier screening at this point is done in the context of the first prenatal visit, when a pregnancy has already started, depriving that couple of the options mentioned earlier. I think that is an unfortunate way to set up a program that is supposed to give people options, not take them away.

Another confusing aspect to all this is that cystic fibrosis is a moving target. This is confusing, but it is wonderful. Cystic fibrosis is every day becoming less and less a life-threatening disease. Protocols are beginning at Michigan, at the National Institutes of Health, and at Iowa to treat patients with cystic fibrosis using gene therapy, where you take the normal gene and put it back into the patient's lungs in order to correct the defect. There is reason for some optimism that some version of this treatment will work over the next five years, and CF will no longer be such a terrible disease. So does it make sense to start screening the population for a disease that may no longer be a disease by the time we get the information back? This is a difficult series of issues to deal with.

Another disorder where a breakthrough is imminent is breast cancer, which affects 11 percent of women. One in nine women in the U.S. will get breast cancer. This is clearly influenced by genetic factors, but until recently we have not had a very good handle on what those genetic factors are. We all know that—if you have a mother or a sister with breast cancer your risk is higher. Very importantly, breast cancer is curable if diagnosed early. One could argue, therefore, that there would be good reason to try to identify individuals who are at very high risk and subject them to intensive surveillance to pick up a cancer before it has spread and cure them of the disease.

We are about to find out who some of those people are. There is a gene on chromosome seventeen which is in the process of being identified. This particular gene is probably carried in an altered form by about one in two hundred women, which makes it about the most common genetic disease. If you are one of those women—the one in two hundred—you have about an 85 percent chance of developing breast cancer and possibly also ovarian cancer by age sixty-five. This is a very badly behaved gene. Furthermore, if you have this gene, you are likely to get breast cancer in your thirties or forties—sometimes even your twenties. This is the most severe end of the spectrum. By narrowing this gene down to a small part of chromosome seventeen, it has already become possible, in families where there are lots of affected women, to make predictions in people in their twenties or thirties about who got the gene and who therefore faces this very high risk.

My point here is to introduce to you the enormous emotional impact that the ability to identify individuals at risk for these conditions is going to have—and is already having in a few test cases. One woman, for example, having seen one sister die of breast cancer and with a second sister just having been diagnosed with bilateral breast cancer, decided that she could not stand living under this cloud any longer. She came into a breast cancer clinic seeking a prophylactic double mastectomy as the only way that she saw of escaping this almost certain death sentence. As it happened, the week she came to the clinic was the same week we completed our analysis of her family to figure out who got the altered chromosome—and she did not. What had started as a research project suddenly became a moral imperative to tell this woman her situation as she contemplated going through radical surgery. We informed her that based on the genetic analysis it appeared she did not inherit the gene, and therefore her risk of breast cancer was no greater than if she were not part of this particular family. As you can imagine, she was elated. She went back and told the rest of her family what had happened. The next day the phones started ringing off the hook because everybody else wanted to know their status too, quite rightfully. We spent hours and hours over the next few months counseling members of this family about their situation.

One woman in the family had concluded that she was not at risk because she was not that closely related to any of the other women in the family who had had breast cancer. Because we discovered her father had been a carrier of the gene and she had inherited it, however, we had to tell her that her risk factor was 85 percent. At age forty, she was immediately anxious because she had not gone through much surveillance. Two hours later she had a mammogram which showed a lesion that was subsequently biopsied. When it was shown to be cancerous she underwent a simple mastectomy and is probably cured. This is likely the first instance where genetic testing of this sort has saved a life from breast cancer.

Two or three years from now, it may be possible for anybody who wants that information to come in and have such a DNA test done to find out whether they carry a mutation in this gene. Of every two hundred women who are screened, one of them will be found to have the mutation. Then we will be struggling with the options about what to do. Intense surveillance would probably be beneficial. Some women would probably choose the option of a prophylactic mastectomy, as horrible as it sounds, because that is generally the safest route to go to avoid the cancer. This is representative of the kinds of dilemmas this sort of testing allows us, yet I do not want to question the value of doing the testing. This sort of testing will probably save thousands of lives over the next ten or twenty years. By identifying the individuals at risk—they are at risk anyway; the test does not make them at risk—we allow them to discover their cancers while they are still curable, thus allowing them to live longer and happier lives. This is particularly appropriate for breast cancer because there is something you can do. If you were simply going to tell those people, "Well, you are at very high risk for breast cancer and there is not a thing we can do about it," I suspect not too many of them would want the information. As Sophocles wrote, "It is but sorrow to be wise when wisdom profits not." One would like the wisdom to be profitable, and I believe if the knowledge offers you options that you can do something about, then you have profited.

All of these issues, as brought up in some small way by cystic fibrosis and breast cancer, but which will be relived with many other conditions in the next few decades, are very much on the minds of those directing the Human Genome Project. In fact, the Human Genome Project has set aside some five percent of its total funding, which amounts to the largest single investment in ethical research in the history of mankind, to try to investigate these issues. What is the possibility of abuse of this information? What about confidentiality? What about discrimination against individuals found to have genetic abnormalities? Will they lose their insurance? Will they lose their employment? I think we all feel intrinsically that one should not be discriminated against on the basis of genes, something about which we have absolutely no choice. At this point there are not adequate safeguards in place to protect against that.

There are a number of other ethical issues—many of them, in fact—that arise from this project. A very important one is the issue of the impact on reproductive decisions. To what extent will this information be used by couples who are choosing what kind of child they want to have?

Jumping ahead to, say, the year 2020, the Genome Project will be completed. We will know about those hundred thousand genes. We will have identified the genetic basis of all single-gene disorders and many other more complex ones. You will be able then, at the age of eighteen, when you are old enough for informed consent, to go to your doctor and say, "I would like to have my DNA checked to see what I am at risk for so that I can plan accordingly." Your doctor can draw your blood and send it off to some massive genetics company. You will then get a report card that tells you what they found. The report card probably will have hundreds of entries on it, but it might include some of the following: a list of conditions that are inherited as recessives, like cystic fibrosis; a series of conditions inherited as dominants; and a much longer list of things we call polygenic, where there are a lot of different genes that contribute, such as the common diseases of cancer and heart disease and diabetes. This is the way that medicine is going to shift into a more preventive mode, instead of treating diseases that are already full-blown. We all say that is what we want. We say that is how health care costs are going to come down. A lot of people are not quite sure how to bring it about. Genetic testing has a lot to offer in that regard, because it allows you to identify who is at risk and treat things before they get out of control.

Suppose, however, you were doing that same test and it was not on an eighteen-year-old who came in for voluntary testing. In this case it was being requested by a well-heeled couple who wanted to be sure that the child they were expecting had the maximum possible genetic endowment. Suppose they got the result back that said the child would be a CF carrier and would have a high risk of colon cancer. These characteristics are perfectly compatible with a very productive life, but would this couple be tempted to say, "Well, maybe we ought to try again." That is a little chilling.

If you think couples would not be likely to do that, and I would have sort of guessed they would not, you might want to examine a special issue of *Newsweek* magazine with a special section called "Made-to-order Babies."[1] It contained a report of a still-unpublished survey done by a group in New England. They asked parents, "What would cause you to want to abort a pregnancy?" Only one percent said they would abort on the basis of not getting the sex they wanted. Six percent said they would abort a child likely to get Alzheimer's in old age. But 11 percent would abort a child predisposed to obesity. We will probably understand the genetic basis of obesity within the next ten or fifteen years. Will couples choose to use this information in that sort of way?

We are clearly going to be struggling with the issue of the gray zone between diseases and traits. I do not believe, and I do not think the American public—even the nonreligious public—believes that the utilization of this technology for trait selection is appropriate, yet there is nothing in place to prevent that at the present time. There is nothing to stop sex selection. I think one of the major challenges that faces society in the next five years, before this technology becomes fully formed, is to decide to what extent this requires oversight—legislation or regulation. Or should we just let this whole process go on in a willy-nilly fashion? I would argue that would be most unfortunate. That kind of debate is going to be difficult, requiring input from the church and all other segments of society, and input by people who are willing to invest in understanding the issues. I challenge you to get involved in those debates. The ethical, legal, and social issues program of the Human Genome Project is actively trying to get such dialogues going, and trying to prepare for the onslaught of technological possibilities.

Lest you be concluding, after hearing the chilling side of this, "Why are we doing this? Why are we spending all this money on this project that has all these possible outcomes?" I cannot emphasize strongly enough, while it has potential misuses, the point of this project and the clear outcome of this project is going to be beneficial to very real people who are suffering from very real diseases.

An eight-year-old girl with cystic fibrosis wrote this charming entry in her diary on August 25, 1989, the day the cystic fibrosis gene was cloned: "Today is the most best day ever in my life! They found a gene for cystic fibrosis." She certainly understood the promise that finding this gene held for her future. That promise is already being realized with the development of gene therapies for CF. That will be repeated over and over again for other diseases. We certainly cannot hold those people hostage to concerns about potential misuses. However, we have to take the responsibility to be sure those misuses do not occur.

Copernicus had his own struggles about the perceived conflict between science and faith. He said: "To know the mighty works of God, to comprehend His wisdom and majesty and power, to appreciate in degree the wonderful working of His laws, surely all of this must be a pleasing and acceptable mode of worship to the Most High, to whom ignorance cannot be more grateful than knowledge." Let us all dedicate ourselves to that principle.

Endnotes

[1]Geoffrey Cowley, "Made to Order Babies," *Newsweek* Special Edition: *The 21st Century Family,* Winter/Spring 1990.

Genetic Promise
and Problems

By C. Ben Mitchell[1]

In general, I celebrate the remarkable advances in genetic science that have marked the latter half of this millennium. I am extremely hopeful that the Human Genome Project will be successful in its goal of mapping and sequencing the human genome with a view toward discovering cures for genetically linked diseases.[2] That advances in genetic science have outstripped our ability to work through the moral and ethical implications of the "genetic revolution" is very troubling to me, however. I am heartened by the foresight of the National Institutes of Health and the Department of Energy in their support for discussions of the ethical, legal, and social implications of the project (often described as the "ELSI component"). The scientific and academic communities are quite rigorously engaged in discussion.

However, apart from a conference held in Houston,[3] a few scattered articles in relatively obscure religious journals, and a lone theologian on a conference panel here or there, little space has been given to discussions of the religious dimensions of genetic issues. Several denominations have adopted statements or resolutions on genetic technology, including a very comprehensive statement by the United Methodist Church.[4] Southern Baptists have yet to examine the issues thoroughly and systematically. Most Southern Baptists know something about the explosion of genetic technology as it is reported in the popular media, but few seem to have given attention to the concommitant explosion of ethical issues relative to the technology.[5] What I hope to do in this chapter is to facilitate thoughtful reflection on several areas of critical concern; namely, prenatal screening, genetic discrimination, and workplace screening and monitoring, offering what I believe to be some prudential judgments about these topics as they relate to the broader subject of genetic science.

Prenatal Screening

Presently, there are two major types of genetic screening tests. On one hand, prenatal screening, the most common application of genetic screening technology,[6] "is aimed at the early recognition of affected individuals in whom medical intervention will have a beneficial effect for the affected individual and/or the patient's family."[7] Examples include prenatal tests for Down's syndrome and neural tube defects. Increasing numbers of prenatal genetic anomalies will be diagnosable by means of genetic screening in the future.

On the other hand, carrier testing is done in order to identify individuals who are at risk of transmitting genetic diseases to their offspring. Screening for Tay-Sachs disease and sickle-cell anemia are classic examples of this form of genetic screening.

As John A. Robertson, Thomas Watt Gregory professor of law at the University of Texas at Austin, has pointed out prophetically,

> Through at-risk or population screening, persons will be able to learn their carrier status for heterozygote genetic diseases, and avoid conception of offspring with undesirable genetic traits. Prenatal, and eventually even preimplantation, diagnosis of embryos and fetuses will permit women to avoid carrying such offspring to term. As new carrier and prenatal tests emerge, genetic selection of offspring characteristics will become increasingly routine.[8]

A major ethical concern, for evangelical Christians in general and Southern Baptists in particular, is how genetic screening will impact the practice of abortion. Presumably, abortion would not be considered in cases in which the diagnosed disease is treatable. But, as Nancy Wexler and others have pointed out, we must "keep in mind that more often than not, diagnostic information will become available well before the ability to act on it therapeutical-ly."[9] Through genetic screening, then, parents will be enabled to predict (with more or less accuracy) whether their children will be affected by a deleterious gene, but will be impotent to do anything about it except have the baby or abort her. The parents of such a child may, in fact, be encouraged to abort the child, (in the language of the psychologist) "due to the anguish of carrying a fetus with a severe or lethal genetic disease"[10] or (in the language of the lawyer) as an expression of "the woman's liberty interest in avoiding pregnancy."[11] Strong social pressures may also be applied to women to abort their "defective" babies so as not to "pollute the gene pool" or "use up valuable medical resources" caring for a baby with relatively low "quality of life."

We must not trivialize or underestimate the anguish involved in having a child with a radical congenital deformity or lethal disease. Human, and especially Christian, compassion demands our utmost concern and care for the parents of children who are devastated by such an event. At the same time, we should not, in my view, condone or support technologies which encourage or are complicit with nontherapeutic abortions.[12]

Most Southern Baptists are committed to the sanctity or sacredness of human life. That is, because of our religious conviction, rooted in the Scriptures of the Old and New Testaments, we believe that all human beings are created in the image of God and are invested by God with sacredness or unique value (Gen. 1:26-27), and therefore, believe that abortion, except to save the life of the mother, is morally repugnant.

Southern Baptists are on record for their over decade-long opposition to abortion on demand and for their opposition to "the use of federal funds to encourage, promote, or perform abortions except to save the life of the mother."[13] Moreover, Southern Baptists are on record as opposing "the testing, approval, distribution, and marketing in America of new drugs and technologies which will make the practice of abortion more convenient and more widespread."[14]

Genetic screening for diseases for which there is no treatment or cure, it seems to me, cannot but lead to the more widespread practice of abortion. In fact, as genetic research continues to offer more sensitive and reliable tests and as increasing numbers of genetic diseases are detectable, decisions to abort affected babies will also no doubt increase.[15] As David Suzuki and Peter Knudtson have observed, "Until effective treatments become available, such tests can offer little more than scientific guidance to inform the decision of parents who are willing to consider abortion to prevent the birth of a child who could be gravely ill."[16]

There are future scenarios in which parents might be pressured to abort their baby if they discovered the baby had a genetic disease. Suppose a program of national health insurance were created. Would it be argued under such a program that it is not in the best economic interest of societal health care for "defective" infants to be born whose care would consume valuable and scarce medical resources?

As a society, we have already travelled some distance down the road toward this kind of "quality of life" ethic. As Marque-Luisa Miringoff says in her important book, *The Social Costs of Genetic Welfare,*

> In the pursuit of good health, we have begun to tread a fine line in "human selection." We often choose to rule out certain diseases or, more accurately, certain human beings with those diseases. In some cases, as with Tay-Sachs disease, an as of now invariably fatal illness in early childhood, such a decision may be motivated by compassion. From many viewpoints, there is little quality of life in any sense traditionally understood, and great anguish and tragedy.
>
> Other diseases, however, challenge our logic more severely; our sense of balance between cost and benefit is not clear. Huntington's chorea is a case in point. Would a Woodie Guthrie be born today? Would his parents, as carriers of this disease, bear a child with the known risk? Could we now or soon screen him out prenatally? If the pace of genetic intervention continues, such an individual would not be born. Yet I, for one, am glad that he lived, although I mourn the anguish of his later life. One wonders, too, whether some perception of his coming illness contributed to the extraordinary creativity of his life.
>
> Clearly, it is a just and meaningful desire to prevent fatal and debilitating diseases. Yet in pursuing this goal, we pay unobserved costs. In eliminating individuals with unwanted diseases, we also create a mind-set that justifies the process of human selection. We thus move into the questionable arena of human worth, and to some degree eugenic thought. We forego the idea of therapeutic change (i.e., dietary change or other forms of treatment) and opt instead for elimination.

Individuals are seen as flawed. It is easier and more desirable to prevent their existence than to work for their survival.[17]

Only a "sanctity of human life" ethic will prevent our society from tumbling down the slippery slope into a holocaust of mandatory abortions and eugenics. Quite apart from abortion, genetic screening for diseases for which there are no treatments or cures also carries unknown psychological risks. For instance, what would be the psychological impact on parents who know there is a high probability that their son will suffer the ravages of Huntington's disease, a terribly painful and finally lethal disease, in middle age? What would be the psychological impact on the son who learns in his late teens that this is the case? How will this impact his medical care?

Other questions regarding prenatal and carrier screening abound. What about the ethics of screening for the purpose of sex selection?[18] How can we be certain the most accurate and valid tests are being used? Who will have access to the test results? What about genetic counseling? Will everyone have access to the necessary *nine* sessions of counseling for Huntington's?[19] Who will pay for the screening and counseling (at $3,000 to $4,000 per test[20])? What about cultural differences between populations?[21] Will affected children routinely sue their parents for "wrongful birth" if they choose to carry them to term rather than abort them after it has been determined that the parents are carriers of a genetically linked disease?[22]

I essentially agree with Professors Bouma, Diekema, et. al., at Calvin College who say,

> Where there is a safe and accurate test for a condition and where the test is related to available and effective treatment, we celebrate this new power to diagnose newborns, children, and adults. Where such conditions are not met, we are more cautious than celebratory, and we are particularly concerned about the sort of mentality that would routinely screen for conditions for which there are neither accurate tests nor effective therapy. We are especially worried about the possibility that people who will eventually suffer from the onset of effects of a genetic disease will suffer the stigma of that disease even before the symptoms become apparent because others know that they are diseased and have a "genetic defect."[23]

Until we know more about the ethical, psychological, and social impact of prenatal and carrier screening, screening for genetic diseases for which there are no cures or treatments should be prohibited or, at least, highly regulated.

Genetic Discrimination

Troy Duster, professor of sociology at the University of California at Berkeley and himself an African-American, observes that "Several important gene disorders tend to overlap racial or ethnic groups. Since these racial and ethnic groups, in turn, are stratified, genetic screening programs are now forced to confront socially sensitive issues."[24]

The history of humankind is littered with horrific examples of discrimination based upon race, creed, and other individual and class distinctions. The history of genetics is not without its own horror stories. The eugenics movement in the early part of this century called for involuntary sterilization of many persons considered "feebleminded," "indolent," and "licentious." By 1907, Dr. Harry C. Sharp, physician to the Indiana State Reformatory, "had performed vasectomies on four hundred and sixty-five males, more than a third of whom were said to have requested the operation."[25] (Presumably, the other two-thirds were done involuntarily!) The State of Iowa passed a law in 1911 that permitted the sterilization of inmates for a variety of reasons, "including drug addiction, sexual offenses, and epilepsy."[26]

Across the Atlantic, in Nazi Germany, the Eugenic Sterilization Law of 1934

> compelled the sterilization of people who suffered from diseases that were alleged to be inherited (including schizophrenia, epilepsy, blindness, and some physical deformities), followed in 1939 by the euthanasia of institutionalized patients with mental and physical disabilities, [which] was justified on the grounds that the public could not assume the expense entailed in maintaining "lives not worth living."[27]

May the world never forget that the most infamous eugenic experiment to date resulted in the attempted extermination of an entire race of people. Hitler's vision, out of which the Holocaust emerged, was fueled by images of genetically "pure" Aryan supremacy.

More recently, we can recall our own history of mandatory sickle-cell screening among African-Americans and what some have called the resultant "public policy disaster."[28] By 1972 at least a dozen states had passed legislation mandating sickle-cell screening. Social stigmatization and discrimination were based upon the results of those tests. As late as 1980, an African-American student was refused admission to the Air Force Academy because he was a sickle-cell carrier (he did not have the disease, but was merely a carrier), despite the fact that there has never been conclusive evidence that one's sickle-cell carrier status poses any risk to the individual.[29]

Even someone of the stature of Nobel laureate Linus Pauling could escape public censure by a culture enamored with the possibility of eugenic technology:

I have suggested that there should be tattooed on the forehead of every young person a symbol showing possession of the sickle-cell gene or whatever other similar gene, such as the gene for phenylketonuria, that has been found to possess in a single dose. If this were done, two young people carrying the same seriously defective gene in single dose would recognize this situation at first sight, and would refrain from falling in love with one another. It is my opinion that legislation along this line, compulsory testing for defective genes before marriage, and some form of semi-public display of this possession, should be adopted.[30]

While this may sound ludicrous to us today and while we might wish to think that we are in some way superior to our forebears, to Hitler, and to the sentiments of Pauling, perhaps we are not. In fact, a biblical anthropology which takes the nature of human sinfulness seriously informs us that we are as susceptible to such heinous thoughts and deeds as anyone in history. To realize this is the case, we need only to be reminded that, in 1988, China passed legislation prohibiting the marriage of mentally retarded persons unless they were sterilized.[31]

Miringoff has pointed out that genetic reductionism (the notion that all social ills can be cured by gene therapy) has fostered social discrimination and runs the risk of devastating the less advantaged of society:

. . . investments in expensive technologies divert attention from social efforts that offer specific benefits for the less advantaged. A significant example lies in genetic screening for mental retardation. Trisomy 21, or Down's syndrome, is of course widely dispersed along the social hierarchy. Yet scientific evidence, accumulated over several decades, consistently demonstrates that genetic impairments account for most upper- and middle-class retardation, but are the source of much less retardation among the lower classes.

In the lower classes, retardation is often a result of poor prenatal care, denial of sensory stimulation, lead poisoning, or a failure of the schools. In short, it is a *social* product. But the increasing use of genetic screening and counseling emphasizes only genetic fallibility and therefore highlights only a portion of the problem. If we continue to address retardation solely as a genetic aberration, we will systematically ignore thousands who suffer the social, not genetic, disability.[32]

Southern Baptists have a rich history of opposition to racism and discriminatory practices. We were the first denomination to support the 1954 Supreme Court decision against segregation in public schools. We observed our first annual Race Relations Sunday in 1965. For well over half a century we have sought to help our constituency fight bigotry and discrimination and celebrate human diversity. In a 1989 resolution, adopted in Las Vegas, Nevada, we affirmed, among other things, our belief "that all people are created in the image of God and are therefore equal." Moreover, we affirmed "our intention of standing publicly and privately for racial justice and equality."[33]

Even though Southern Baptists have not yet specifically spoken to the issue of genetic screening, it is relatively simple to translate our abhorrence of racism to an abhorrence of all forms of stigmatization and discrimination against individuals based upon genotype. Arthur Caplan, director of the Center for Biomedical Ethics at the University of Minnesota, has said, "The world has been worse off for human genetics and its application to particular groups."[34] One may be assured that Southern Baptists will do all we are able to ensure that Caplan's historical reflection does not become a future reality.

The Genetics, Religion, and Ethics Project of the Institute of Religion and Baylor College of Medicine in Houston, Texas, issued a "Summary Reflection Statement" on the Human Genome Project. The June 1, 1992 statement is apropos:

A religiously based consensus on the full and equal dignity of all human persons is often contradicted in practice by discriminatory prejudice of one group against another. Ethnic and racial diversities among human beings are due in large part to genetic factors which must never be interpreted as indices of personal

or social worth. Neither should the presence of physical
or mental disabilities, whether or not they are due to
genetic inheritance, detract from one's personal or
social value.[35]

The statement goes on to point out that,

Because the Jewish and Christian religious world
view is grounded in the equality and dignity of individual persons, genetic diversity is respected. Any move to
eliminate or reduce human diversity in the interest of
eugenics or creating a "super strain" of human being
will meet with resistance.[36]

With respect to genetic screening the statement says, in part,

Religious values mandate the defense of personal
privacy, integrity of the family, and good social relations. Therefore, they support policies and methods of
securing consent to have access to genetic information
obtained through screening. Moreover, the use of confi-
dential information must be carefully circumscribed to
avoid embarrassment, social stigmatization, disruption
of marital and familial relations, and economic discrimination. Care should be taken to avoid or prevent the
unjust uses of an individual's genetic data in respect to
securing and holding employment, insurance, and
health care.[37]

In light of the discussion above, I argue that because the information discovered by genetic screening is so personal, private, and
sensitive, individuals should have a legal right: (1) to know the
information gathered by screening, (2) to know when genetic information is being gathered, (3) to refuse or consent to give such
information and/or order that such information be destroyed.

Also troubling is the fact that because genetic science is still in
its infancy, and because genetic tests are becoming increasingly
sensitive, no one knows, today, all that may be revealed by genetic
screening tomorrow. Not only must presently available genetic
information be protected, but future information must be protected
as well. As Holzman has argued, "Regardless of how many refuse
testing, society's imposing its will on them may exact a greater
price in tearing our social fabric than caring for their affected offspring."[38]

Workplace Screening and Monitoring

Concerns about the implications of genetic screening by
employers and insurance companies are well documented.[39] As the

interest in screening for drugs, and now HIV, has grown, so has the interest in the genetic screening and monitoring of employees. Rationales for the genetic testing of workers are numerous, according to the Council on Ethical and Judicial Affairs of the American Medical Association.

In some cases, there may be an argument in favor of testing for public health reasons. Companies have expressed concern about the possibility of an employee's genetic susceptibility to illness from exposure to a chemical or other substances in the workplace. In addition, employers may not want to hire individuals with certain genetic risks for jobs that bear on the public's safety. Other justifications are based not on concerns about health but on concerns about costs, specifically costs to the *company* of hiring workers with a genetic risk of disease. Individuals who have a heightened risk for certain illnesses may be less attractive as employees; on average, they may be able to spend fewer years in the work force, and they may impose greater health care costs on the employer.[40]

It will be useful to make a distinction between genetic screening and genetic monitoring. Genetic screening tests may be used to identify individuals who may be hypersusceptible to certain occupational hazards, such as industrial chemicals, air pollutants, or manufacturing materials. A person who "fails" the test, presumably, would be denied employment. Genetic monitoring tests may be used to detect genetic damage to workers who are exposed to (what might be to them, at least) hazardous materials.

An incident reported in *Scientific American* provides an interesting case study:

A graduate of a police academy in the Midwest was about to be hired as a policeman when it became known he had a family history of Huntington's chorea, an incurable disorder that causes physical and mental degeneration in middle age. The man was told he would have to be tested for the gene causing the disease before he could be hired.[41]

This case is riddled with questions. Would the discovery that the man was a carrier for Huntington's exclude him as a potential candidate for the job? What kind of genetic counseling would he be offered? How many persons will know his status? Will the record of his status follow him? Is the police department responsible for the results of the test, since a percentage of those who learn they have the gene for Huntington's commit suicide? If he were hired despite his status as a carrier, would he be refused insurance even though he is asymptomatic? What if his test results were false-positive? Who decides which genetic illnesses should be targeted?

Early statistics indicate that many (perhaps most) persons who are at risk do not wish to be tested for genetic disorders. Wexler observed that although there is a population of 125,000 Americans at-risk for Huntington's disease, only about 1,000 individuals worldwide had requested testing by fall of 1992.[42] She goes on to point out that "the current linkage test is necessarily complicated and time-consuming. The testing process can take a year or longer; total costs run to $3,000 or $4,000."[43] Questions about who pays for lost job time and testing are not easily answered. With scores of different tests on the horizon and increasingly scarce medical resources, whether or not we ought to offer tests for diseases without cures is no "ivory tower" issue.

It should be pointed out, of course, that conducting genetic screening and monitoring in the workplace may be in the employer's best interest. Employers have a legal responsibility to protect the health of their employees. Through genetic screening employers might be able to "weed out" those employees, or prospective employees, who may later become expensive liabilities under existing health insurance, disability, and worker's compensation programs. The AMA's Council on Ethical and Judicial Affairs opined, "Employers may not want to hire individuals with a predisposition for cancer, Alzheimer's disease, or other illnesses since these individuals might impose higher health costs on the employer."[44] Additionally, through genetic monitoring, employers or government agencies may better be able to detect and relieve the deleterious health-related impact of various pollutants in the workplace. As Suzuki and Knudtson point out, we might be able to look on these workers "as warning beacons representing the final boundary beyond which society should no longer condone further environmental contamination."[45] Genetically monitored workers may become the human equivalent of the canaries used in the past to detect the presence of gases in mine shafts. At what price progress?

Social justice issues and issues of rights and duties have not been easy for Americans to work out. It may not be overstating the case to say that genetic screening and monitoring in the workplace are potentially the stuff of which civil wars are made. Extreme caution must be exercised, ethical issues thoroughly scrutinized, and problems thoughtfully and sensitively solved, before wide-spread employee testing takes place.

The Americans with Disabilities Act will, no doubt, help resolve some of the issues at stake in genetic screening and monitoring. But most researchers tend to agree that additional legislation will be necessary to protect against discriminatory practices in the workplace.[46]

Taken to a gloomy extreme, obsessive genetic screening of employees could one day even result in a Huxleyan hierarchical caste system of workers. The lowest rung of the ladder would be occupied by those whose genetic test results marked them as hypersusceptible workers, stigmatizing them as economic untouchables destined to be chronically unemployed. At the highest rung would be workers whose test results established them as model employees whose genotypes—genetically resistant, in one way or another, to the environmental or psychological stresses of important occupational tasks—would guarantee them permanent, if monotonous, positions in the work force.[47]

Conclusion

It is too early to know whether the information discovered through the Human Genome Project will catapult us into the Brave New World or the New Dark Ages. Sadly, we will not know the outcome until after the fact. We are optimistic about the results of the project because we believe that all truth is God's truth. At the same time, we are realistic in our view of the propensity of human beings to use good things for bad purposes (evangelical Christians call this propensity the sin nature). This propensity is clearly part and parcel of every human being despite the fact that, at least to date, no genetic cause for the "illness" has been found.

The psalmist declares that human beings are "fearfully and wonderfully made" (Psalm 139:14). I celebrate the Human Genome Project and the effort to understand more completely just how wonderfully constructed we are. I am extremely hopeful that many genetically linked diseases will become curable as a result of the project. But because of our gloomy history of abusing genetic information and because "the technologies underlying new genetic screening tests have improved so rapidly that they have already far outpaced our ability to interpret their results,"[48] I maintain that every effort should be made to prevent genetic screening from being used for the purpose of elective, nontherapeutic abortions, as a means of discrimination, and/or as a violation of worker privacy. We must resist premature legislation which could jeopardize an informed, public debate on these issues and declare our support for legislation which protects the value and dignity of individual human beings.[49]

Endnotes

[1]The substance of the concerns expressed in this chapter were first delivered in public testimony before the Institute of Medicine's Committee on Assessing Genetic Risks in Washington, D.C., September 17, 1992.

[2]*Understanding Our Genetic Inheritance, The U.S. Human Genome Project: The First Five Years FY 1991-1995* (National Institutes of Health Publication No. 90-1590, April 1990).

[3]Sponsored by The Institute of Religion and the Baylor College of Medicine and supported by an ELSI grant and The Episcopal Church Foundation, the Genetics, Religion and Ethics Conference met twice: once in 1990 and again in 1992. Between national conferences working groups met to formulate documents which sought to address a variety of issues from a religious perspective.

[4]Some denominational statements include a report from The General Convention of the Episcopal Church adopted in July 1991; pronouncement on The Church and Genetic Engineering by the Seventeenth General Synod of the United Church of Christ, adopted in 1989; a 1987 statement on genetic engineering by The Church of the Brethren; and the substantial document offered by the United Methodist Church Task Force on Genetic Technology.

[5]It could be argued that there are no *new* ethical issues raised by genetic engineering. Every new technology brings with it its own set of potential dilemmas and conundrums, most of them relevantly similar to the ones we have faced already. Similarly, the Human Genome Project probably presents few, if any, novel ethical issues. What the burgeoning genetic technology does present, however, is a venue for nearly all of the dilemmas that face the entire realm of the biological sciences in one neat (or perhaps not so neat) package.

[6]David Suzuki and Peter Knudtson, *Genethics: The Clash Between the New Genetics and Human Values* (Cambridge, Mass.: Harvard University Press, 1989), 166.

[7]Thomas D. Gelehrter and Francis Collins, *Principles of Medical Genetics* (Baltimore: Williams and Wilkins, 1990), 271.

[8]John A. Robertson, "Procreative Liberty and Human Genetics," *Emory Law Journal*, Vol. 39, No. 3 (Summer 1990), 697.

[9]Nancy S. Wexler, "Disease Gene Identification: Ethical Considerations." *Hospital Practice* (October 15, 1992), 145. Gelehrter and Collins point out in *Principles of Medical Genetics* that, "Screening tests are an essential part of standard medical care and are generally directed at early diagnosis of *treatable* diseases" (emphasis added). This, of course, raises the question of whether or not we should routinely screen for diseases for which there are no treatments or cures.

[10]Gelehrter and Collins, 282.

[11]Robertson, 713.

[12]I would define "therapeutic abortion" here as one which is necessary to save the physical life of the mother.

[13]*Resolution No. 2—On Sanctity of Human Life,* adopted by the Southern Baptist Convention meeting in Atlanta, Georgia, June 4-6, 1991.

[14]Ibid. The sentiment of this portion of the resolution was clearly directed at drugs such as RU-486, the French abortion pill.

[15]Screening may lead to sex selection abortion or be used to fashion so-called "designer babies" whose genotypes correspond to a parental menu of desirable attributes.

[16]Suzuki and Knudtson, 166. Also see, Theodore Friedmann, "Molecular Medicine," in Bernard D. Davis (ed.), *The Genetic Revolution: Scientific Prospects and Public Perceptions* (Baltimore: The Johns Hopkins University Press, 1991), 143.

[17]Marque-Luisa Miringoff, *The Social Costs of Genetic Welfare* (New Brunswick, N.J.: Rutgers University Press, 1991), 159-160.

[18]"In India and Asia it is already becoming common for pregnant women to seek tests of the fetus to determine its sex. Female fetuses are frequently aborted. In these cultures, girl children are much less valuable than boy children. Girls and women are in fact considered not much more valuable than many animals—certainly less valuable than a healthy water buffalo. Female infanticide has long been common, and aborting a female fetus little more than a temporal extension of this practice." Joel Davis, *Mapping the Code: The Human Genome Project and the Choices of Modern Science* (New York: John Wiley & Sons, Inc., 1990), 263.

[19]See Wexler, 147.

[20]Wexler, 148.

[21]Miller and Schwartz argue that before genetic services are offered to at-risk populations, cultural differences need to be understood. The cultural impact of genetic screening must be

investigated more thoroughly before it is offered widely. Cf. Shelley R. Miller and Robert H. Schwartz, "Attitudes Toward Genetic Testing of Amish, Mennonite, and Hutterite Families with Cystic Fibrosis," *American Journal of Public Health,* Vol. 82, No. 2 (February 1992), 236-242.

[22]The notion of assigning "blame" for genetic disease must be studied more carefully. The popular media are powerful tools in shaping public *mis*perceptions. For instance, consider the following recent headline, "Tracing genetic ills to grandma," *USA Today,* July 31, 1992, 1-D.

[23]Hessel Bouma III, Douglas Diekema, Edward Langerak, Theodore Rottman, and Allen Verhey, *Christian Faith, Health, and Medical Practice* (Grand Rapids: William B. Eerdmans Publishing Company, 1989), 245.

[24]Troy Duster, *Backdoor to Eugenics* (New York: Routledge, 1990), 37.

[25]Daniel J. Kelves, *In the Name of Eugenics: Genetics and the Uses of Human Heredity* (Berkeley, Calif.: University of California Press, 1985), 93.

[26]Ibid., 100.

[27]Neil A. Holzman, *Proceed with Caution: Predicting Genetic Risks in the Recombinant DNA Era* (Baltimore: The Johns Hopkins University Press, 1989), 224.

[28]Duster, 45.

[29]Thomas F. Lee, *The Human Genome Project: Cracking the Genetic Code of Life* (New York: Plenum Publishing, 1991), 278-279.

[30]Cited in Duster, 46.

[31]Jody W. Zylke, "Examining Life's (Genomic) Code Means Reexamining Society's Long-Held Codes," *Journal of the American Medical Association*, Vol. 267, No. 13 (April 1, 1992), 1715.

[32]Miringoff, 68.

[33]*Resolution No. 2—On Racism*, Adopted by the Southern Baptist Convention, meeting in Las Vegas, Nevada, June 13-15, 1989.

[34]Zylke, 1715.

[35]*Summary Reflection Statement*, Genetics, Religion and Ethics Project, The Institute of Religion and Baylor College of Medicine, The Texas Medical Center, Houston, Texas (Houston: The Institute of Religion, June 1, 1992), 2.

[36]Ibid., 4. Unfortunately, we are, as a society, only now coming to appreciate biodiversity and the interrelatedness of all living

things. Some argue that we have come to appreciate it too late. Could the same be said for genetic diversity?

[37]Ibid., 5.

[38]Holzman, 229.

[39]And again, the popular press is shaping public opinion on these issues. See, for instance, Shannon Brownlee and Joanne Silberner, "The Age of Genes," *U.S. News & World Report,* November 4, 1991, 64-76.

[40]"Use of Genetic Testing by Employers," Council on Ethical and Judicial Affairs, American Medical Association, *Journal of the American Medical Association,* Vol. 266, No. 13 (October 2, 1991), 1827.

[41]Tim Beardsley, "Fatal Flaw: Who will have the right to examine your genes?" *Scientific American*, Vol. 265, No. 6 (December 1991).

[42]Wexler, 147.

[43]Ibid., 148.

[44]"Use of Genetic Testing by Employers," 1828.

[45]Suzuki and Knudtson, 175.

[46]Zylke, 1716.

[47]Suzuki and Knudtson, 171.

[48]Ibid., 170.

[49]See *Summary Reflection Statement,* Genetics, Religion and Ethics Project, 6.

It Matters Where You Start

By Kurt P. Wise

Our experience tells us that proper behavior is only possible with a certain minimum amount of knowledge. A child playing in the yard who lacks the experiential information of how moving cars can damage a human body on impact, and/or lacks the ethical information from her parents that it is wrong for her to play in the road, may just do so. A child learning to toddle, who lacks the experiential information that different objects have different stabilities, and/or lacks the ethical information that it is wrong for him to pull himself up on the tablecloth, is likely to pull the coffeepot down on himself (as I did when I was young). The same applies to mankind as we venture into new areas such as genetic engineering, trans-species transplantation, mass family planning, and so on. If we launch into those areas without considering all the information at our disposal and even searching out more information, both scientific and ethical, then we are almost certain to fail to do right.

As we search out information, one very important area of consideration is that of origins. Our experience has taught us over and over that if we wish to understand something completely, we must consider its origin. As a scientist, as I evaluate a particular fossil in the fossil record, I ask such questions as how such an organism came to be and how it came to be found in the rock that it is in, and how it came to get into the shape that it is in, and so on—I evaluate its origin. As a doctor evaluates a person's complaints, he determines what it is that might be the common origin for all the symptoms. We, as parents, as we deal with a sibling squabble, usually seek to determine how it began. As I personally deal with my sin, I determine how the matter began—what was the true sin of attitude which brought about the effect of the obvious transgression. The origin of a matter is essential to a complete understanding of it. In fact, it might be argued that the origin of a matter is one of the most important pieces of information that one should get in order to understand a matter.

The more complete is our knowledge of the origin of an object, the greater and more varied is our understanding of the object. My appreciation for something as unimpressive as garage doors was much enhanced when I worked in a garage door factory and actually took part in the construction of them. As I witnessed the events which took place in the origin of a single section of a garage door—the calculating, the measuring, the marking, the cutting of metals, the riveting of pieces, the cutting of glass, the laying of grommet and insertion of glass—I began to understand a garage door much better than ever before. This is not to mention the many other events which ultimately went into the construction of a garage door, like the mining and refining of ore, the formation and molding of metal sheets, the formation of springs, rollers, rivets, nuts, bolts, and even the machines we used! I can say that not only can I better appreciate the complexity and makeup of a garage door, but I also know better how to take care of a garage door, and better know when the garage door is broken, and even to some extent better know how to fix it if something about it goes wrong. I could still benefit from more knowledge, but knowing some of the events which enter into the origin of a garage door has much enhanced my knowledge of the workings of a garage door, and my ability to use it properly.

Another value to the study of origins can potentially come in the area of teleology. If I understand why something came to be, I not only understand the object better, but I also better know how to use the object, and may better realize how to repair the object if damaged. I can remember watching my father pound nails into a board with a hammer. By watching the process, I quickly came to understand how nails got into boards. And, by watching, I gradually even became capable of duplicating the event—some of the time. Yet, there were times after I had duplicated the process exactly (or so I thought), when I met with disapproval. Truly, I understood how nails came to be in boards, and I understood how to properly get nails into boards, and I had (at least this once) mastered the process of getting nails into boards, but I lacked one very important piece of information. Before I understood why nails were pounded into boards, I could not fathom what was wrong with nailing the cabinet doors shut or nailing the nail-less dining room table, and so on! I came to learn, as most people do, that in order to fully understand what someone is doing, it is often very important to know why they are doing it. When I learned that nails were used to fix two boards together that you wanted firmly attached to each other, that substantially changed how I applied my mastery of nail-pounding. In like manner, an understanding of the origins of an object—both the process of its origin and the purpose of its origin should allow us to better: (1) understand the workings of an object; (2) care for an object; (3) master the use of an object; (4) recognize disrepair in an object; (5) repair an object if it breaks; and (6) know when and why we should utilize an object.

It would stand to follow that as we begin to ask what is right and what is wrong in our pursuit of genetics, a key requirement is that we understand the origin of organisms and their genomes. As we consider what is right and wrong in the manipulation of the genetics of organisms we use as food, and/or those we use as experimental subjects, and/or those we deem pests, we need to consider the origin of the organisms and their genomes. In like manner, as we study the genetics of humans we should seek to understand the origin of humans and their genome. If we understood the process whereby these came into existence and the purpose for their existence, we would be in a better position to develop a proper ethic in their manipulation. We would better know how and when to care for, recognize errors in, and even repair genomes. This chapter will offer only the most introductory of comments on the effects one's view of origins has on ethical decision-making in the science of genetics.

Genetics and Young-universe Creationism

According to Scripture, God is fully responsible for bringing into existence all objects and beings that exist and have existed besides Himself—both those which are material and those which are immaterial (Gen. 1:1; Ex. 20:11; Neh. 9:6; John 1:1-3; Acts 14:15). This indicates that our God is transcendent—that He is in no way dependent upon the physical or spiritual universe. At the same time, it indicates that the physical universe is fully dependent upon God for its origin. Scripture further indicates that that which He created reflects His nature (Pss. 19:1-6, 97:6; Acts 14:17; Rom. 1:19-20) and everything that exists is sustained in its existence by the continual workings of God (Col. 1:17; Heb. 1:3). Thus, not only are all things indebted to God for their origin, but they continue to be dependent upon God for their continued existence, and God defines their purpose. It is because of this utter dependence upon God that we who hold to this view of origins look to God to define absolute morality—to provide the correct ethic. We cannot look to society, or ethics boards, or lobbying groups, or rights activists, or votes, or even ministerial groups to derive our ethic. Our ethic must come from God—from His Word, from His nature, from His Spirit. We also cannot tolerate pluralistic ethics—for there is only one God and thus there is only one ethic.

A Normative Ethic

On the sixth day of His creation, God called all that He had made "very good" (Gen. 1:31)—apparently a pronouncement of both aesthetic and moral purity.[1] That perfection persisted in the spiritual world until the fall of Satan (Isa. 14:12-15) and in the physical world until the curse (Gen. 3:16-19; Rom. 8:19-23). Before the curse, then, all that was in the physical world was as God wanted it. The events and nature of the pre-fall world can then be considered normative, or God's ideal. Since man's sin brought imperfection into the physical world, the correction of known imperfections toward a restoration of pre-fall conditions can be considered a justifiable move toward God's normative. As we understand the nature of the pre-fall world we can place imperatives and constraints on our Christian ethic. As an example, before the fall man had perfect communion with God. The fall of man broke that communion, and we now struggle against the effects of our sin as we strive to restore it to pre-fall quality. Similarly, before their sin there was unrestrained communion and cooperation between Adam and Eve. Now we struggle with many burdens of inter-human conflict. Our imperative, then, is to strive toward a restoration of communion with God and communion and cooperation among men. This is a substantial part of our Christian ethic and is part of what is taught in the two greatest commandments (Matt. 22:36-40).

According to Genesis 1:29-30, there was no carnivory among pre-fall animals. There was also no pain in childbearing (Gen.

3:16), no death (Gen. 2:17; Rom. 5:12, 19), and no thorns (Gen. 3:18). Furthermore, since such things as aging, parasitism, and disease involve physical decay which seems inevitably to lead to death, it can be argued that these arose only after the fall. Since the toil of gardening is due mostly to the growth of one plant (a weed) at the expense of another, and much animal death is due to struggle for survival against other animals, the curse seems also to have introduced competition into the biological world. The lack of pain in child-bearing, the lack of inter-human conflict, and the lack of disease and death as well as the similarity between the pre-fall world and the new heaven and the new earth [tree of life (comp. Rev. 22:2 and Gen. 2:9); no death (comp. Isa. 25:8; Rev. 21:4 and Gen. 2:17); no carnivory (comp. Isa. 11:6-9; 65:22; Hos. 3:18 and Gen. 1:29-30)] would seem to imply that before the fall there may have been no sorrow or pain. It follows, then, that our efforts to fight aging, parasites, disease, weeds, sorrow, and pain may be unconscious efforts to fight the effects of sin and restore us to a pre-fall status. Scripture's weak justification of the fight against disease (e.g., the healings of Jesus, the apostles, and the prophets; 1 Tim. 5:23) seems to underscore the fact that at least some of our attempts to restore pre-fall conditions should be a part of our ethical imperative. This would seem to be a large part of our justification for medicine in general.

At the same time, reason for caution exists in generally applying such an imperative. Parasites have very complex life cycles which seem to be designed expressly for the life of parasitism. It is more than difficult to conceive of such life cycles as imperfections in design. Similarly, the complex design of our nervous system involved in detecting pain does not seem to indicate imperfection. Most organisms have very clever ways to avoid being eliminated in the struggle for survival, and carnivores seem to have been very carefully designed to hunt down and eat meat. Thorns and toxins in plants show evidence of complex design, and bacteria and fungi seem to be specially designed to feed on dead organisms. It would appear, then, that not all of the changes which came about at the time of the fall were imperfections. Some of the changes seem to have been specially designed provisions for the survival of organisms in a post-fall world—perhaps created with the organisms as unexpressed genetic material.[2] In order to punish man for his sin, man was to die (Gen. 2:17), but in order to avoid the accumulation of billions of bodies, bacteria and fungi may have been designed to break them down. In order to punish man for his sin, the ground was to produce less fruit, plants were to become less edible, and man was to work in order to get food from the ground (Gen. 3:17-19). But, in order for other organisms to now get sufficient sustenance for survival, carnivory may have been instituted, and mechanisms to survive in the struggle for survival were provided to them. None of these provisions can then be considered imperfections. In fact, the mandates which indicated that it was good to eat meat (Gen. 9:3; Acts 10:9-16) would seem to indicate that carnivory is not an imperfection at all. It would not be justifiable, then, to restore pain-sensitive nervous systems, the thorns and toxins in plants, the carnivory in animals, and the decomposition activity of bacteria and fungi to a pre-fall state. This, in fact, would do more harm than good to the organisms which possess these traits for their sustenance.

Other changes at the fall, however, can be considered true imperfections. Genetic errors (tens of thousands strong in man), such as mutations and chromosomal aberrations, seem to be imperfections which man would be justified in eliminating in order to restore a pre-fall normative. In addition, many diseases are caused by organisms whose pre-fall roles have changed. Pathogenic viruses, for example, may have been originally "organs" of sexual reproduction for bacteria. Similarly, bacteria and parasites may have been originally free-living organisms in mutual symbiosis with their hosts (e.g., the gut fauna of cattle which allows them to digest cellulose and lignin). After the fall, perhaps due to genetic errors in these organisms, they may have begun to involve themselves with cells and/or organisms other than those for which they were intended. In these cases we may well be justified in dealing with organismal pathogens in our effort to restore pre-fall conditions. However, if this line of reasoning is correct, then it seems that it might be possible to correct the organism's erratic behavior by correcting a genetic error within without having to destroy the organism as a whole. Perhaps this suggests a resolution of the dilemma facing the CDC in Atlanta with regards to what to do with the entire known population of smallpox organisms. Perhaps these organisms should be studied to determine if a correction of a genetic error could result in an organism which could be released—so that an organism would not have to be destroyed.

Pre-fall conditions also put constraints on our activity. If the pre-fall condition is truly normative or ideal, then we cannot consider any change from that ideal—even if perceived as an improvement—as right. There is much interest in genetics to create new and improved genetically engineered organisms. If we truly believe that our Creator knows best how organisms on this earth should interact, and that our Creator is a provider to even the bacteria, then we must accept the fact that the best possible organisms are already programmed into the genetic material of organisms, less any imperfections which have arisen since the fall. Up until genetic engineering, breeding studies have utilized genetic information already programmed into organisms. The different varieties of dogs, for example, were not created by us, they were selected by us. We only chose various combinations of already extant genetic information to produce the dogs we have about us. Early studies in genetic engineering did the same thing, but now we have the technology to create new genetic material, with the express intent of improving organisms. I would maintain that this violates our normative ethic.

The 'Creation Mandate'

In pre-fall time man was given the authority over the earth and the animal world (Gen. 1:28). Never rescinded anywhere else in Scripture, we can consider this pre-fall condition a normative for us and thus should still be a part of our ethical imperative. Yet what does this so-called "creation mandate" mean? Historically, the passage has been used to justify everything from strip-mining to animal experimentation to meat-eating to wiping out of disease and much more. Since much of the discussion centered on this imperative ignores other moral imperatives in Scripture, I feel most of it is invalid. First of all, the passage only gives us explicit dominion over animals in the sea, the air, and the land. Other than the obscure phrase "subdue the earth," it is not at all clear that it has any application to geological resources—before or after the fall. Besides that, since carnivory was nonexistent in the pre-fall world, and disease was probably absent as well, the imperative's meaning in the pre-fall world could not have applied to meat-eating, disease-fighting, or animal experimentation. Since meat-eating was allowed in a separate imperative (Gen. 9:3; Acts 10:9-16) and disease-fighting can be justified in other ways (see above), it is not clear that this imperative refers to those things either.

The passage indicates that Adam and Eve were placed in a position of higher authority than the earth and the animal world. One also gets the sense that man was given the fathership or guardianship of the earth and its creatures. In that sense the application of the passage for today may be that man has been given the authority over the earth and creatures in order to care for them and man. It may be related, then, to the previous discussion. Man can be seen to have the responsibility to look out for the good of the creation—to correct the mistakes that he has been responsible in introducing in an effort to restore the animal world and the earth to pre-fall conditions. It is a bit broader than the previous understanding of the imperative, because it tells us that we have a strong responsibility not just to utilize the earth and its creatures in order to correct the post-fall errors plaguing man, but that we have a responsibility to correct the post-fall errors plaguing animals on this earth and the earth itself. We should not just focus on correcting the genetic load of humans, but should seek to better animals as well. In this sense we cannot justify eliminating types of organisms simply for the sake of man's good. This underlines again the fact that we should probably not just seek to eliminate pathogens, but determine how to restore those pathogens to their pre-fall condition.

The Priority of Successful Development

If one believes the earth is very young, one necessarily believes that God created Adam as an adult. One also believes that many other aspects of His creation were created in a complete or whole form. The sun, the moon, and the stars would have been created as mature bodies, possibly even with light being created between the body and the earth. Trees and flowers would have been created already grown, and streams would have been created already with sand bars and banks and fish already grown. This principle is not without precedent elsewhere in Scripture. Jesus's first recorded public miracle, for example, involved the turning of water into wine (John 2:1-10). In the context, we are led to believe that the change was almost, if not completely, instantaneous and that the wine was mature when made. Likewise, the healing miracles involved instantaneous steps of complete healing. Similarly, when we accept Christ He instantaneously creates within us a new person (2 Cor. 5:17; Rom. 6:6); and at our resurrection He will change us in a moment into a new form (1 Cor. 15:51-52). It appears that it is simply God's nature to create things instantaneously and completely. If this is so, then God's purpose in creation involves the mature organism. Although God creates the genome of organisms in order to produce subsequent generations of the adult forms He desires, His ultimate purpose is not the genome or developmental stages but rather the complete and mature organism. This means that the adult form is normative, with genetics and development being means to this higher end. As a result, any disease or event which prevents maturation or alters development, thus preventing or endangering the production of an adult should be avoided and/or corrected if possible. The correction of maturation-altering diseases would lie under this imperative, and so would abolishing abortion in any form. Furthermore, procedures such as amniocentesis, which endanger the baby but usually serve no constructive function (other than perhaps encouraging the abortion of children), should be avoided.

The Constraint of Kinds

According to Genesis chapter one, plants and animals were created to reproduce "after their kinds" (Gen. 1:11-12, 21, 24-25). What is strongly implied here is that when God created organisms He created a certain number of kinds (some creationists call them "baramins"; others call them "basic types"), where the members of a given kind of organism were not to reproduce with organisms outside their own kind. Once again, this is a pre-fall condition and should be considered a prescription for an imperative. Although we may have the power to cause it, we cannot consider it right to pass genetic material between organisms of two different kinds. There is currently a strong drive to take genetic information from very different types of organisms and combine them to produce an organism with unique abilities. Although this kind of activity uses only available genetic information, and thus does not create new genetic information, it does combine the information in ways never intended. If we are not to improve upon the pre-fall condition, then introducing genetic material which has never been possessed by a baramin before should not be allowed. The biggest challenge in applying this imperative is determining whether two organisms are from the same baramin or not. Only recently have creationists begun to develop methods capable of identifying baramins and their boundaries.[3] Much research will be necessary to resolve most baraminic relationships. On the other hand, certain baraminic boundaries are easily identified. Man, for example, is a specially created being distinct from all other organisms (Gen. 1:26-27; 2:17). All other organisms are outside the human baramin, so genetic information from any other organism which does or did not exist in the human genome should not be placed within humans.

The Warning of Ignorance

As outlined above, it can be argued that God created a significant amount of genetic information which was unexpressed at the time. It is very likely, for example, that pain sensation, the capacity for carnivory, floral thorns and toxins, as well as complicated mechanisms for survival under conditions of competition were pre-programmed for expression at the time of the fall. It is likely that this is just a small part of the latent information placed within genetic systems. For some organisms we have witnessed extraordinary genetic variety. For example, a large number of varieties of dogs, pigeons, pheasants, goldfish, and cattle have been produced from what appear to be uniform wild types. The changes have been too rapid to be due to creation of new genetic information by mutation, chromosomal aberration, recombination, or trans-species viral transmission. The most reasonable explanation would seem to be that the information was already preprogrammed into their genome by God. In like manner early baramin studies[4] indicate that many baramins contain dozens of species. Since most land animal baramins came through the flood via two representatives (Gen. 6:19-20; 7:2-3), the last forty-five hundred years or so since the flood have seen a tremendous amount of diversification within baramins. Again, this diversification is probably greater than that which is possible due to the spontaneous development of new genetic information, and is most probably due to the expression of genetic information latent in organisms which survived the flood.

So whether we are speaking about organisms at creation, at the flood, or even now, we have reasons to believe that organisms possess a lot more potentially useful genetic information than they express at any given time. A substantial portion of the human genome is not used in the production of a human being. Usually this unused information is considered useless. Yet, if most organisms possess unexpressed, potentially useful, but latent genetic information, then much of the unused genetic information may be useful. God's nature seems consistent with this idea as well. God's omniscience allows Him to know all that an organism will experience in the history of the earth. Because of His provisional nature, God may have provided organisms at their creation with all the information necessary to take on whatever forms were necessary for survival in a changing world. God's wisdom gives Him the ability to design organisms with a high degree of integration and complexity—not only the complexity needed for any given time in history but also the complexity for all other times as well. Because of His perfection and efficiency, it seems most likely that God would have provided organisms with only as much genetic information as they needed and no more. All this makes it very likely that unused genetic information is just that—unused—and not useless. If this is true then genomes contain a much higher level of complexity than we currently recognize. As such, our low level of understanding makes our manipulations of genetic material very dangerous. Knowing so little, it seems very improbable that man is likely to improve or correct the mistakes in such a complicated genome. At best we need to proceed with great caution. We should not simply assume that unused genetic material is unimportant to an organism or to the ultimate survival of its baramin.

Preservation of Baramins

God created a number of baramins and then gave man the authority to take care of them. It stands to reason that we should not allow the extinction of any baramin if it is in our power to prevent it. However, since a baramin often expresses itself in a variety of species, this imperative is not equivalent to an imperative to preserve all species from extinction. If a species is threatened with extinction whose genetic information is collectively contained in other living species of the baramin, then excess resources need not be devoted to the preservation of that species. On the other hand, a threatened species which is the only living representative of a baramin should be preserved if possible.

The Racism Condemnation

All humans are descendant from a single couple (Gen. 3:20) only about six thousand years ago. More recently—about forty-five hundred years ago or so—humans were represented by a mere eight people (Noah, his three sons, and their wives). This would be insufficient time to allow human or cultural evolution. Yet, much less time than even that is available, for advanced culture existed very early in earth history (Gen. 4:20-22). It appears that man was created with complete language and cultural ability, so no person or people is more or less evolved than any other. There is also no justification for blaming any racial differences on divine judgment. The most popular example in this area is to identify the black race with Noah's curse on Ham. Yet, Ham's ancestors not only include the blacks, but also the Egyptians, the North African Arabs, the Canaanites, the Philistines, the Sumerians, the Babylonians, and the Assyrians (Gen. 10:6-20). There is no biblical justification for treating any race differently from any other.

Genetics and Other Origins World Views

This chapter has provided a few examples of ways in which one origins world view can impact ethical issues in the area of genetics. Other origins world views impact ethical issues with different conclusions. Some people, for example, feel that God was/is not involved in the origins and/or sustenance of anything. These people are deists or atheists. Others feel that we and the universe are god or at least part of god. These people are pantheists. Neither of these groups would appeal to God's Word for their ethic, nor necessarily believe that there is an ethic. Rather, any desired ethic would best be derived by collective human decision. The answers on any of the issues discussed in this chapter are not only likely to be different, but to differ from one sub-population to another, and even from one time to another within the same population.

Even theistic creationists, those who believe that God is transcendent and involved in the creation and sustenance of the universe, differ on a variety of other issues. Some creationists, for example, consider the first chapters of Genesis so symbolic that God's original creation did involve disease, suffering, pain, sorrow, toxins, aging, carnivory, physical death, thorns, parasitism, and competition. The original creation cannot be considered normative and therefore attempts to combat aging, parasites, disease, weeds, sorrow, and pain must be justified in other ways. There may also be no reason to believe that pathogenic organisms were ever non-pathogenic, so there is no necessary reason to restore and preserve them. Furthermore, if God brought and brings organisms into existence by means of mechanisms which caused a net improvement in organisms over time, then there is no real reason to discourage attempts to improve organisms. In fact, these attempts could be seen as ways to meet ends which God has in mind.

Creationists who feel that God produced most, if not all, organisms by modifications of an original organism will not consider trans-specific genetic transfer to be inherently wrong. They will also feel differently about the importance and methods of species preservation. They will also feel differently about the inherent complexity of genomes and thus be less concerned about the manipulation of genetic material in general.

Conclusions

One's view of origins has a profound effect on one's ethic—including one's ethic in the field of genetics. Because "small" differences in origins world views have large differences in ethical implications drawn from them, it is critically important that Christians very carefully consider what their views on origins are. I would suggest that those views should be drawn carefully from Scripture, with a priority given to the words of Scripture and the physical data of the physical universe. Neither the theories of man drawn from Scripture nor the theories of man drawn from the physical creation should hold priority over the words or works of God. Models of origins should be critically and minutely tested against all of Scripture and all known data of the physical world.

I believe in a transcendent Creator and sustainer God who is the prescription of the only true ethic. I believe He created the original earth about six thousand years ago with a variety of optimally designed organisms, providentially containing latent genetic information to be useful to the organisms in their present and for their future. The complexity of the genetic material of these organisms so far exceeds our understanding that we must be very cautious as we manipulate genetic material. I also believe that God created a certain number of distinct kinds or baramins, the genetic material of any one of which should not be crossed with that of any other. I also believe that man's sin brought a number of changes into that originally perfect creation. Some, such as carnivory, pain sensation, and survival mechanisms were probably expressions of created latent genetic material. Others, such as mutations and chromosomal aberrations, pathogenic behavior, and aging are physical imperfections permitted into the creation. Correction of these imperfections toward restoration of the pre-fall normative condition is justifiable, but the improvement of genomes over the pre-fall condition is not. Because I feel that man has been given the authority to care for the biological world, it is our responsibility to correct genetic mistakes in organisms and to preserve baramins (not species) when it is in our power to do so. In my view of origins racism is completely unjustifiable and such things as abortion and unjustifiable amniocentesis are wrong.

Christians should be proactive in developing a solid ethic on all issues. We should provide answers to questions which scientists and others are not trained to answer. In order to do this, I think origins scientists, philosophers, and biblical scholars with a common commitment to the truth of Scripture and creation should combine their efforts toward that common goal.

Endnotes

[1]James S. Stambaugh, *Death Before Sin?* Impact Article 191:i-iv, 1989 [found in *Acts & Facts* 18(5)].

[2]For more discussion see James S. Stambaugh, "Creation's original diet and the changes at the fall," *Creation Ex Nihilo Technical Journal* 5(2), 1991, 130-138.

[3]Walter J. ReMine, "Discontinuity systematics: A new methodology of biosystematics relevant to the creation model," 207-213,

and Kurt P. Wise, "Baraminology: A young-earth creation biosystematic method," 345-358, in *Proceedings of the Second International Conference on Creationism, eds. Robert E.* Walsh and Christopher L. Brooks, (Pittsburgh: Creation Science Fellowship, 1990). See also Siegfried Scheven, *Typen des Lebens,* (Studium Integrale, Pascal-Verlag, Berlin, German: in press), and Kurt P. Wise, "Practical baraminology," *Creation Ex Nihilo Technical Journal* 6(2) 1992, 122-137.

[4]Wise, 1992; Scheven, in press.

The End of the Autonomy Road

By Thomas Elkins

Medicine is problematic because people are problematic. I wish everything were black and white, but sometimes it simply is not. There are times when it is a puzzle.

We have a very active Christian Medical and Dental Society at Louisiana State University where I teach. We had a very active one at the University of Michigan. We try to get across to others that the Bible still counts. It is a Book you can read and can depend upon. Even when things tend to be bothersome and beyond our understanding, it is a Book to return to.

I would like to mention some verses that I think about often. Then I want to share what ethics means to me as a physician in my area and relate some of my personal story.

Matthew 25:31-32 says, "When the Son of man shall come in his glory, and all the holy angels with him, then shall he sit upon the throne of glory: And before him shall be gathered all nations: and he shall separate them one from another, as a shepherd divideth his sheep from the goats." Later in this familiar passage Matthew lists the many things we can do to meet human needs and suffering. Finally the Lord is asked, "When saw we thee a stranger, and took thee in? or naked, and clothed thee? Or when saw we thee sick or in prison, and came unto thee? And the King shall answer and say unto them, Verily I say unto you, Inasmuch as ye have done it unto one of the least of these my brethren, ye have done it unto me" (Matt. 25:38-40).

As we look at issues such as genetic counseling and prenatal screening, think back on that term, "the least of these," and what it means in your own setting. It has taken on different meanings around our house over the past few years.

I also think often of John 9:1-3: "And as Jesus passed by, he saw a man which was blind from his birth. And his disciples asked him, saying, Master, who did sin, this man, or his parents, that he was born blind? Jesus answered, Neither hath this man sinned, nor his parents: but that the works of God should be made manifest in him." Finally, I would like to remind you of one other simple, small verse, Romans 3:23: "For all have sinned, and come short of the glory of God."

When we talk about biomedical ethics, we are not talking about philosophic ethics. We are not talking about the theories of ethics or the principles of ethics. But we are, in a very real sense, talking about narratives, about stories, about ethical concerns as they deal with the lives of people, because these are what make it biomedical ethics. These are what make it clinical. These are what make it useful and meaningful. So I would like to share one of those stories, a story that deals with amniocentesis, a story that deals with sex selection, and a story that deals with my own growth and development and change within our own household.

Amniocentesis represents, in my mind, the changes in the technologies of choice in prenatal diagnosis over the past twenty-five to thirty years in the United States. We have experienced a tremendous boom in prenatal diagnostic technology. We used to talk in terms of amniocentesis—where we stick a needle into the amniotic fluid around the baby *in utero,* withdraw some of that fluid, and analyze it—as being a wonderful tool of technology in which we could not only make prenatal diagnoses, but many times we also could use that tool to tell whether a baby was mature enough to deliver late in pregnancy, or to tell whether an infection is present that would require us to act suddenly to even save the baby's life. We found out that amniocentesis was a wonderful window to see what was going on *in utero* so that we as physicians might respond more appropriately.

Then there came a time when it appeared that we could also diagnose a vast array of genetic disorders and other types of disorders *in utero* through the methodology of amniocentesis. Today that is almost rudimentary technology in prenatal diagnosis. Now we talk in terms not only of amniocentesis, but chorionic villi sampling, where we take a needle and sample the tissue of the placenta itself early in pregnancy. We talk in terms of ultrasound that is so much more diagnostic today than it once was. When we compare the ultrasound we use today to what we used ten and twenty years ago, it is almost like the verses in Corinthians that talk about once seeing through a glass darkly and now seeing clearly (1 Cor. 13:12). What we thought was clear twenty years ago seems like a dark glass today because we can tell so much difference in terms of what is happening *in utero*. Now we are actually talking in terms of serum testing, where we can simply draw blood from the mother and tell very much about what is happening *in utero* with the fetus. So there have been changes in technology.

There also has been an evolution in terms of issues and ethical principles throughout these twenty to twenty-five years in terms of the growth of prenatal genetic counseling. These issues perhaps are best exemplified by sex selection, because it is the first of the issues that brought a challenge to the whole concept of autonomy as an unlimited principle in our country.

There also has been a development of character and understanding within our own family that mirrors, I am sure, the same type of growth and development that has happened in many other families. As you begin to learn and to understand, God gives you gifts in life you did not expect, and you begin to respond in ways that you never thought possible.

My story begins in 1983. I had just returned to the United States from about a five-month stint in Africa with the Southern Baptist Foreign Mission Board. This was the third such stint that my wife and I had done. Each trip always gives us a different viewpoint. We come back to America somewhat puzzled by Americans. We go and spend our time with some of our wonderful physicians, nurses, and evangelists who work in the rural parts of West Africa, and we come home and are saddened oftentimes by what we see in our own country. This was one of those times, because when you leave the Third World, you leave an ethic that is simple, that is understandable, that is not problematic in many ways because it is an ethic of vast need, an ethic of desperation, an ethic of beneficence where people are hoping and praying for bits of kindness. It is an ethic of justice, where people are crying out that things have been wrong, things that can be corrected many times in ways that seem easy and apparent. It is an ethic of caring, where people desperately care for one another for the simplicities of life. But it is also an ethic of joy and of gratitude when you do achieve some of life's most humble possessions.

Then we returned to the United States, where we faced an ethic of wealth, an ethic of contentment, an ethic called choice where people have choices. They have choices of what they are going to wear every day. They have choices of what television shows they are going to watch. They have choices of what video they want to rent that afternoon. They have choices of what church they want to attend or even if they're going to go. They have choices of what college they want to attend. They have choices of what teachers they want to sit and listen to if they choose to go to college. They have choices of who they marry. They have choices of whether they even want hot or cold water running from a faucet. All these are things we don't see in the Third World.

I returned in 1983 to participate in a conference sponsored by the American Law and Medicine Society in Boston entitled, "What About the Children?" The gist of the conference was a discussion of new reproductive technologies and where we in America fit in that discussion. It was aimed mainly at surrogate motherhood, which was a major issue at that time. It is an issue that has come and almost gone in our society, but for a while it blazed across the headlines of almost every newspaper in our land.

There was one speaker at that meeting that I won't forget. She was the leader of an international organization for women's rights, and she came to say to that group that for the first time women in the world were realizing that there was something beyond the absoluteness of autonomy and choice in terms of prenatal diagnosis. Her organization had taken a stand internationally against sex selection as a choice for women to make in prenatal diagnosis. The reasons were quite clear. Over 99 percent of the time this test was being used internationally, it was to eliminate female fetuses in countries such as China and India. She said this was no longer a reasonable use of technology. Here was a person who stood for choice but now said that there is a time when choice is not an absolute and when we must stand and say, "This does not make sense. This needs to stop."

I thought that was an amazing comment, and it generated a great deal of concern at the conference. The conference presentations were supposed to become a book, and, of course, it didn't. That message seemed to dwindle away, and over the next few years we heard over and over about sex selection. Amniocentesis grew to become a major industry, and then offshoots of amniocentesis began to grow as well.

Growth and change come to families, too. The year 1985 was a year we will remember around our house. We changed jobs, going from the South to Michigan. It was also a time when my wife came to me one day in the hallway of our home and said, "It has taken me six years, but at this point in time, if we had a chance to do it all over again, I would not want any three children other than the three I have, including the middle one." I said, "That's quite an admission." Now, you have to understand: our middle one is a character; our middle one has Down's Syndrome. But my wife had come to the realization after six years that, given our choice—not God's choice, but our choice—she would want no other child, including that middle one. That implies something that is called coping, which we in the United States don't do very well.

If you look for textbooks on how to cope, you won't find many because they are not written, and those that are written are not written well. You might go to something that is at least commonly quoted, though it is hard to find, a book by a social worker named Beatrice Wright.[1] She listed how we should cope with each other and how we should cope with people in our society who are different.

She said, first of all, you have to devalue physique. That is hard for Americans to do. We are a "billboard culture." We get up every morning, and we love to see how each other looks. We spend at least forty-five minutes to an hour making sure we look okay before we leave the house. But that is America. Yes, one of the major problems we have is learning to devalue physique, to look at each other and to recognize that our inadequacies are us and that is okay.

The second thing we have to do is isolate the disabilities within us. Because one has a particular disability or handicap does not mean that as a person he or she is disabled or handicapped. I am overweight and ugly. Those are particular disabilities. Some may have a problem speaking or hearing. Some may have a problem with fine motor functions; others may have headaches or almost daily PMS. These do not mean that any of us are evil, bad, wrong, or worthless persons. These mean that some of us have a particular disability or handicap.

Third, we also need to learn to redirect goals. I never intended to be where I am at this point in my life. In fact, I never intended to be at LSU. We had it all planned to be medical missionaries in Africa. It was a goal we wanted badly. When we left Baylor

College of Medicine and spent the first year after medical school in Africa, we were sure that was what the Lord had planned for us. To be honest, my wife and I have looked at our lives as sort of failures ever since that point. But He gave us some children that keep us in this country, and we had to redirect our goal. We had to redirect some of our lifestyles because of the people that we are and the "disabilities" in our midst. To cope, you have to begin to do that.

And finally, you have to learn to change comparative values to asset values. One of the things we do as parents is love our children. The problem is that sometimes we Americans only really love our kids when they do well, and we forget to love our kids when they don't. One of the biggest problems we have as Americans is wanting to be excellent all the time and hesitating to love that child who can't be, won't be, or shouldn't be. It is difficult becoming a parent and learning to love until you have a child with a disability who looks you right in the eye and says with her actions, "Hey, this is all it's going to be, Dad." Now figure what that means. "This is all it's going to be." We can get Ginny out and run around the block for four years, but she is not going to win any 100-yard dashes. But she is happy with that, and when the race is over, she is jumping and shouting, "Me won!" And we have begun to be winners, too. But it has taken a while. It has taken that changing of comparative values to asset values. We no longer care if our kids make As, Bs, or Cs in comparison to my cousin's kids or the kids at church, or the kids in the next block—but it has taken a while to reach that point. We as Americans have had to learn to cope.

By 1985 we were finally beginning to cope around our house, and some things were beginning to make sense. That was about the time of a conference at the University of Michigan on fetal sex selection. The conference started by focusing on the medical need to have fetal sex selection done occasionally. There are those illnesses, some of them quite severe, that are genetically transmitted in a sex-selected fashion. Hemophilia is one, but the list is actually quite long. So people could make a very rational argument for having fetal sex selection as a use for amniocentesis and, at that point in time, chorionic villi sampling. This discussion was actually fairly heated, because some of the women's rights activists at Michigan also had read *The New York Times* and knew this was still being used in developing countries throughout the world to eliminate female fetuses, and they were quite irate about that. So this again was an interesting discussion during the conference, but that sort of died there.

In the fall of 1991 I heard another treatise at the University of Michigan by a very learned philosopher on fetal sex selection. This time I finally realized that this argument was one that was not going to leave Americans because we could distort anything, and we would distort this one as well. Many people may have read in seminary the book, *Historians' Fallacies*.[2] That textbook discusses logic and analysis and reason and how we can make arguments which are fallacies in their very beginning, but by making those arguments so well we can convince people of a totally different point of view. That learned philosopher did that extremely well that day. He spent almost an hour proving to all of us in the room that if we did have a male-dominated world, we would not necessarily self-destruct because of overt violence. Once he had proven that, he then said that fetal sex selection, even if it weeded out women, would be fine. Now, if you can follow that, you are much better than I am. But I thought as I walked out, the length of absurdity to which we will go as Americans is sometimes impressive. At the bottom of this man's argument was that concept of autonomy which has been something we as Americans have gone back to again and again.

In biomedical ethics we talk in terms of theories and principles and normative values. Now principles have usually been listed as things such as beneficence, truth-telling, justice, nonmaleficence, and autonomy. Autonomy has been the overriding principle of biomedical ethics in the United States since the early 1960s. However, it does appear to have some limitations. That was something you almost could not admit in the 1960s, 1970s and early 1980s.

Autonomy actually has a short history. Most people see autonomy as stemming from those Bill of Rights issues in the 1700s in our country, or from the English Magna Carta and other rights issues by which our country was founded. But it does not go back much farther than that in medicine, unlike beneficence, unlike justice, unlike nonmaleficence, which go back to Hippocrates and even before in the history of medical ethics. Autonomy is a fairly recent principle, as principles go.

We have begun to realize that there are intrinsic and extrinsic limitations to the concept of autonomy. But these realizations have come slowly. Today, if you subscribe to a number of ethics journals, as many of us in medicine do, we now read constantly how people are realizing that there are limits to a person's autonomy. But that was never said in the 1960s and the 1970s. You simply would not read it in any journal talking about ethics. In fact, autonomy was held so strongly to be the overriding ethic, that beneficence—that is, the will to do the good for someone—was equated to paternalism in articles and, therefore, denied as a reasonable principle.

We now realize that autonomy does have some limits, although they may be few. It is a value only for self, in many ways, that is derived from one's own thought and intellect, so therefore it has limits that it places upon itself. It has no ultimate moral qualities, no sense of goodness beyond self-worth or self-value, depending on the clarification of one's own values. Autonomy lacks something called humility and gratitude. When some of the scholars of ethics were asked how Christian ethics fits into secular ethics today, they said that without Christian ethics, secular ethics is powerless to act. Their reason was that Christian ethics interjects into secular ethics the concepts of humility and gratitude. Without those concepts, you have no reason to want to act. You have no reason to want to respond in an ethical way.

One of the major problems in autonomy, though, is that it ultimately is not very open to other views that may conflict with itself. Oftentimes when we are on ethics committees today, if we look around the room and see that everyone there has a strong pro-rights view, or pro-autonomy view, we kind of get a chill, because we know the meetings are going to be loud, harsh, and fast, and oftentimes we are going to leave wishing that we had more time to discuss an issue that people simply will not allow to be carried any farther. It is a rights orientation. It may be any kind of rights— pro-choice rights, pro-life rights, pro-disability rights, pro-women's rights. We physicians often feel closed out of those discussions. It can be a totalitarian conservatism that does not allow us to even place an individual patient into a discussion that may make a difference, or it can be a totalitarian liberalism that looks at us and simply says, "Listen, either get as liberal as we are, or get out." We as physicians are left looking at this crowd of people they call an ethics committee and wondering what we're supposed to do with the patient after they've left the room. That is the intrinsic limitation of autonomy.

But there are extrinsic limits to autonomy as well. Autonomy does not encourage ethical discourse, working toward a consensus of opinion based upon recognized societal goals and norms. It recognizes no "good" that we can all agree upon. Anything that someone would say is good is liable to be contradicted by the ultimate person who believes only in autonomy by their viewpoint of good, which may be totally different and often self-defeating. We have seen that the extreme of autonomy can lead people into doing things that even become harmful. Sex selection is a good example, where women's rights activists who were totally pro-autonomy-oriented went to such an extreme that they finally had to say, "This is not so good" and "Stop." We have seen it now with adolescent sexuality, where people who were totally for freedom of sexual expression have finally moved from an era of sexual revolution and sexual freedom into an era of sexually transmitted diseases. They have said to themselves, "Some of this is not so good," and they have begun to back up some. We have seen it in issue after issue where autonomy has reached its limits and actually has resulted in America turning upon itself.

Perhaps the biggest problem with autonomy is that it reduces health care to a technical field. It reduces it to consumers and providers. No longer do you have people with a covenant response to each other, a people who are caring for one another. You have, instead, one person expressing strong desires and rights and noticing how those are limited by contract, and another person responding and offering within the limits of that contract and rarely beyond. This also has been part of the legacy of autonomy in our society. Furthermore, it does not motivate us to help others in a very strong way in a time when we are facing worldwide epidemics and problems.

An article in the *Journal of the American Medical Association* about three years ago stated that the ethic of autonomy in the United States was not strong enough to push doctors to treat patients with AIDS. If you think about it, it is not. It is an ethic that will make us double-glove and wear glasses and wear something resembling a space suit to do surgery, but it will not push us to care for an AIDS epidemic that may outgrow even our abilities to care for it.

Autonomy also denies rights to those who can't express them. If you can't tell someone what your autonomous rights are, you have very little chance in the United States of having those rights respected. We tried very hard to get this point across in the Baby Doe discussions. They are still arguing it, saying that surrogate discussions of rights can oftentimes be as acceptable as persons expressing their rights themselves. But carry it on out to the time when you will be elderly and unable to express what you would like to have done with yourself, and you begin to sense the worry and fear that an ethic that is based only on autonomy will bring to our society.

In 1990 a book came out by Dr. Edmund Pellegrino called *The Restoration of Beneficence in Health Care.*[3] It was a wonderful book because it gave a history of autonomy in our society and then said there are limits that we now must realize, and we must look back at why we want to care for one another and why we really want to have health care at all. It is not the economics of it that drives us to want to provide health for each other. It is a genuine will to want to do good for each other and see each other grow in a community with a sense of commitment for one another. All of these things seem to make sense.

Then in 1992, as the story continues, I was at a National Association of the Society for Pediatrics in Adolescent Gynecology, a meeting held in Nashville, Tennessee, where they explained the newest type of genetic screening now available to Americans. We are not talking amniocentesis now. That is only a part of things. They weren't even talking chorionic villi sampling. They were referring to doing serum tests on mothers and looking at particular kinds of hormones and then putting those together in a computer and telling you who is at risk to have a child with Down's Syndrome. It was called the triple screen for Down's Syndrome. It involves a serum test for alphafeta protein, a serum test for estradiol, and a serum test for human chorionic gonadotropen, usually called HCG. You put these three tests into a computer formula, and you can come out with a risk factor that basically is equivalent to the risk factor a woman faces at age thirty-five for having a child with Down's Syndrome. Now for the past twenty years we have found it acceptable in America, in general terms, to offer amniocentesis or chorionic villi sampling or whatever they would want to do for testing to a mother who is age thirty-five or over to detect fetal anomalies. There are more anomalies detected than Down's Syndrome, but that was always the most prominent one. So what our scientists have now done is figure out a way of mathematically arriving at this same risk factor. So now they wanted to put this test to an entire population of people of all ages and see how worthwhile it would be.

At the University of Tennessee in Memphis, they tested 2,067 teenage pregnancies. The cost of that was not small. They found one Down's Syndrome fetus. As the researcher presented this paper, which was named the prize paper of the entire convention, she presented the paper very proudly, but she was immediately asked, "Do you think this was cost-effective? How much did this really cost?" She told about the cost, and then she said, "Why, yes, it was certainly cost-effective. The fetus we found was terminated." Those words hit me very hard. I was the moderator of that session, and it took everything I could do not to stop the session and ask them about the ethics of what they were doing. I closed the session rather quickly and after talking to this person, found that this was part of an entire process they had been undertaking for the past two years at the University of Tennessee. They presented their next paper a few months later, entitled "Triple Screen for Down's Syndrome," looking at all pregnancies of women under age thirty-five. They used 8,431 pregnant women, and this time found four fetuses with Down's Syndrome. Three, however, were missed. At that point in time we finally said, "We need to find out what you are doing and why," because, for some reason, this was incredibly bothersome to me. I was a physician who had been in OB/GYN for a long time. We had offered the tests to women for a long time, but it didn't seem so bothersome as this, and I began to ask why. What price is too high a price for our society to pay for the concept of choice? How high a price will we pay for the autonomous right for people to choose?

The simple market price of those tests gets staggering. It costs about $40 to $80 to have the serum test done in Tennessee. At our own institution at Michigan, it costs about three times that much. The ultrasound required for those who are in the high-risk group is about another $100 to $300 per pregnancy. The amniocentesis is about another $500 to $1,500 to top off the risk group to see if you really have a fetus with Down's Syndrome. The overall price for finding one fetus with Down's Syndrome is between $106,000 and $300,000 per fetus found. This is incredibly distressing to me because what is not mentioned are the untold amounts that will follow because the test does not find every fetus. Therefore, as soon as the laws are in place, those missed will result in malpractice suits, which will raise the price tremendously. We are talking in terms of millions of dollars. These costs are much, much more than any one of us as Americans ever thought would happen in our society as we chased down fetuses with Down's Syndrome.

But there was also a price to be paid in integrity. When I went to the American College of OB/GYN annual meeting, I found several industrial booths marketing with big signs: "Triple Screen for Down's Syndrome—Detect and Find Down's Syndrome in a New Way." They were all written in a delightful style. They had wonderful artwork. They were very colorful. I went up to the executives of one of these companies, and I said, "You know, those tests you are marketing also find many disorders that you know are much, much more serious and lethal than Down's Syndrome. Why are you marketing this for Down's Syndrome?" The guy looked at me like I was an idiot, and he said, "It sells. Americans know what Down's Syndrome is. They don't know a lot of those other things very well. It sells," and he turned around and walked off. We are willing now in America to be even dishonest if "it sells,"and that is something I am having trouble swallowing even today. That is our marketing industry, which pays for many of these tests and many of these experiments to be done.

We challenged the researchers to give us a cost analysis that said this was really cost-effective. So they quickly pulled out some old literature, and they put in a cost analysis for a person with Down's Syndrome. Now you and I might have thought they would have instead thought back to, "Do the new ways of testing reduce ultimately the number of necessary amniocenteses?" which could be cost-effective. Would it reduce the number of potentially harmful events for a fetus *in utero* if unnecessary tests were done? That would be cost-effective. Ninety-nine plus percent of tests done for women in pregnancy are negative in genetic screening, so many women have a positive benefit from being screened in that they are no longer anxious, they feel much better, and they have a security about their pregnancy that they didn't have before. That would have been perhaps cost-effective. But what they chose to do for a cost-effective analysis was to put a dollar figure on the person with Down's Syndrome. They listed basically higher health care costs, social work and counseling, increased divorce rates, decreased productivity of parents, problems with siblings. All of these things, they said, indicate that a person with Down's Syndrome costs $196,000 in a lifetime. What a disastrous amount. I can't think of a physician who has been through medical school, residency, and probably some post-doctoral fellowship who doesn't cost all of us at least two or three times that amount. I don't know how many other people have cost society a tremendous amount with their own educational efforts and experiences. The cost figure was presented in a vacuum. I have a feeling many of our own kids will cost us that much or more before it is all over. And yet, we decided that $196,000 for someone with Down's Syndrome was not acceptable, and so, therefore, that person should be hunted down *in utero* and prevented from entering our society.

The analysis was not only presented in a vacuum, but it was untrue and noncontemporary. It ignored the progress made in persons with Down's Syndrome over the past twenty years. The

thing it ignored most was the fact that people such as those with
handicaps like Down's Syndrome can have a tremendous benefit
on our society. We often think about burdens versus benefits. It
has become an ethical norm in medicine. We must analyze the
cost of what we are doing to a "burdens-versus-benefits" philosophy. We in America can tabulate burdens very well. We know
exactly how much each burden costs. But no one can tell you anything about benefits. It is very difficult to put a dollar sign on a
person and say that your benefit has been $50 in the past day,
even if you are a salesman. But we have chosen to do that in order
to justify genetic screening for people with handicapping disabilities.

When they chose Down's Syndrome with which to do this, they
made a poor selection. No other group in our society has changed
so much in terms of its prognosis over the past fifty years. In the
1930s and 1940s we talked in terms of a person with Down's
Syndrome living nine years. We now talk in terms of their living
beyond age fifty-five unless they are one of the less than 1 percent
that have an uncorrectable defect *in utero* and are born in a way
that we can't usually fix. There are very, very few of them with a
particular heart defect. No other group has been able to achieve
the educational growth that group has had in special education
and now normal school education over the past thirty to forty
years. We used to talk in terms of 50 to 70 percent of people with
Down's Syndrome being severely and profoundly mentally retarded. We now talk in terms of less than 5 percent of that population
being in those IQ groups. In fact, the vast majority of people with
Down's Syndrome now have an IQ of between sixty and seventy,
which makes them mildly to borderline mentally retarded.

We used to talk in terms of people with Down's Syndrome
being in institutions, and now very few are in institutions. Most of
them are in our communities. We now talk in terms of supported
employment, and we see them in the workplace and our everyday
environment. What we are not talking about, though, are the benefits they give to us. From them we learn that we all are limited,
that we have our own abnormalities, our own disabilities, and our
own dysfunctions. We learn that the term "normal" is fragile and
probably false. From them we learn that we can experience joy in
the most mundane and simple of things, such as putting two fingers together. You never thought that would be a problem, until
you worked with a child with Down's Syndrome for years picking
up pennies, until finally they could do it with those two fingers.
Their excitement overflows as they jump up and down on both feet

and shout to you with the "thumbs up" sign, "Me won!" Then you realize how simple life can be and yet how exciting.

We begin to learn not only joy but patience and perseverance. We begin to learn those age-old concepts that we often have forgotten, things called unmerited love, unconditional favor, the Christian concept of grace. When we talk about eliminating these people from our society, those are the things we're talking about eliminating. It is not that we are eliminating someone with a handicapping disability. It is that we are eliminating from each of us the spark of understanding, of our own limitedness, and yet in a strange way, our own capacity to give and to love. That's what we're beginning to eliminate in the United States.

As we talk about the entire situation of genetic counseling in America, some things are becoming obvious. The professional community, of which I am a part, is pushing this genetic technology, yet often knows absolutely nothing about the people with the genetic disabilities for whom they are screening. One of the recommendations we are making is that from now on anyone who does genetic counseling be required, at least for some part of their professional career, to work with people who have developmental disabilities.

We are asking in a time when our government, our people are saying that we want social diversity, that we look to the professional community and say, "This is something you must also protect."

We do not want to create a society in which all deviations from the norm have been screened out, and then, when we have made that society, ultimately discover that "normal" was an illusion. So we are asking them to back off and to look instead for their technologies to be used in more reasonable and sensible ways. They are saying, "Yes, but we must use it in some ways, so how?"

Over the next ten to fifteen years we as Americans will find usefulness and disuses for genetic screening and genetic technologies. For many people, it will not be a black and white issue. Many people would like to see these screens used to prevent certain situations which can be terribly tragic in life: to find an encephali *in utero* and to allow that pregnancy to be stopped; to find the fetus with Tay-Sachs disease and allow that fetus to be stopped before a life of terrible suffering that is terribly brief ensues. There can be those settings in which it is not black and white, but when we carry it too far, and when the cost of choice becomes higher than any of us ever imagined, we must have the capacity to stand and say no. We must be able to draw a line

157

somewhere in the sand and say, "Past this point we will go no farther."

Endnotes

[1]Beatrice Wright, *Physical Disability: A Psychological Approach* (1960).

[2]David Hackett Fischer, *Historians' Fallacies: Toward a Logic of Historical Thought* (New York: Harper & Row 1970).

[3]Edmund Pellegrino and David C. Thomasma, *For the Patients' Good: The Restoration of Beneficience in Health Care* (Oxford University Press, 1988).

PART III
Crisis at the End of Life

Dying Well: Death and Life in the '90s

By Gary E. Crum

Euthanasia is popularly referred to as "mercy killing," or sometimes as the bringing about of an "easy" death. It is at the center of a public and private debate that covers a wide range of ethical and religious dilemmas, and is the subject of many a treatise and late news "think piece."

It has been increasingly in the forefront in part because of a general decline in our willingness as a society to leave life and death decisions to the medical profession, which has dealt with these questions for centuries; and in part because modern medical science has provided us with new options/decisions about maintaining life in the face of terminal illnesses and advanced physical deficiencies that would have killed us quickly in past decades.

With more decisions to be made and with less willingness to allow physicians to oversee these decisions for society, biomedical ethics dilemmas such as euthanasia have become issues that lay men and women routinely scrutinize. Issues before the voters in some West Coast states have tried to make it legal for doctors to give some patients a fatal overdose of drugs (none have passed yet), and one country (the Netherlands) currently has what is, in effect, a court-sanctioned national policy permitting doctors to do this.

Most of us cannot reach middle age without having to face the question of the medical "aggressiveness" we wish to see taken in regard to the treatment of an elderly relative. Questions of life and death—abortion, genetic engineering, the patient's right to refuse care, euthanasia—seemingly become more common with each advance in medical technology.

Attending these changes has been an increasing public interest in examining suicide and assisted suicide for the dying. Derek Humphry, of the pro-euthanasia Hemlock Society, advocates suicide in some cases and has even published a book available in many public libraries about what drugs to use to kill oneself and what steps to take to be successful.[1] He sets the scene for this advocacy with the following scenario:

> You are terminally ill, all medical treatments acceptable to you have been exhausted, and the suffering in its different forms is unbearable. Because the illness is so serious, you recognize that your life is drawing to a close. Euthanasia comes to mind as a way of release.[2]

According to Betty Rollins, writing the foreword to Humphry's book: "Some people want to eke out every second of life—no matter how grim—and that is their right. But others do not. And that should be their right."[3]

Euthanasia Terminology and Advanced Directives

Philosophers and theologians sometimes divide the topic of euthanasia into subcategories based on whether death is seen more as an act of omission or commission. It is called "active" euthanasia when death is the result of some overt action—such as giving to another or taking yourself an overdose of drugs in order to avoid a "harsher" fate. It is called "passive" if death is hastened by the omitting of some expected action, such as the refusal to place a patient on a drug that might be expected to prolong life for some limited length of time.

Euthanasia is also referred to as voluntary or involuntary, based on whether the person whose death is being hastened has expressed support for the action. Since euthanasia is seen by some as a benefit even when it is involuntary, it carries with it the assumption that the action is in the best interests of the person whose death is hastened (see the case study of Karl Brandt). If the person has expressed a desire not to be subjected to euthanasia, then the subsequent hastening of death, if not homicide, is at the least extremely paternalistic to the point of denying true personal autonomy.

Finally, euthanasia can be categorized as being "self-administered" or "other administered." A person who gives herself an overdose of drugs to hasten death is considered to have undergone self-administered euthanasia, or to have committed suicide. Someone who has, for instance, asked his relative to shoot him and put him out of his misery has undergone other-administered euthanasia. Obviously, self-administered euthanasia is always voluntary.

In reviewing passive euthanasia, the question comes up about "extraordinary care." This phrase refers to the medical and ethical judgment that a certain type of care is beyond the care expected, given the likelihood of benefit to the patient. This could be because the care is experimental and not known to be successful, or, in the euthanasia debate, it is because the patient is unlikely to benefit from the extra hardships this care will bring in terms of prolonged suffering and/or high medical bills. The emphasis here is not so much on the medical care being rendered as it is on the patient's condition, since one patient might routinely be given care that would be considered extraordinary for another. For example, hospitals and nursing homes have policies for establishing "no code" or "do not resuscitate" (DNR) orders for patients. A DNR order might be given to a patient with three terminal illnesses who is close to death and who has been given cardiopulmonary resuscitation several times. Meanwhile, CPR would be given as routine care to another patient who had no terminal illness but had a reaction to a new drug and went into anaphylactic shock.

Another phrase sometimes encountered that sounds like "extraordinary care," but which is different, is "artificial treatment." This phrase is found in some "living wills"—statements of your wishes in case you become incapacitated and unable to express yourself to caregivers. By saying you do not want any "artificial treatments" you are not just excluding what might be extraordinary care, you are denying yourself a much larger set of care options. This is particularly important if you have signed a living will that does not take effect until after you become terminally ill. Similarly, if terminal illness is not defined, especially in regard to the expected life span before natural death, or if that life span is not a short time of, say less than a week, the living will might have consequences that you do not anticipate in shortening life that you would like to live.

Living wills, contrary to popular opinion, in most states do not allow you to avoid pain and suffering from an illness. They are instead designed just to reduce the medical options. Unless those medical options happen to be prolonging your life, your pain and suffering will not be affected. However, in the final stages of life when pain control may be needed by some patients, drug dose levels may reach a level that could, as an indirect effect, shorten life.

Most states have passed some kind of "advanced directive" legislation for living wills. The directives in your state might also include "durable powers of attorney." These directives designate a person whom you choose to make your treatment decisions if you are unable to so yourself. Unlike the living will, the durable power of attorney allows someone you trust the legal authority to review the specific facts of your case after you have reached some extreme situation. This person then acts according to what he or she knows your values and wishes would be. In states that do not have advance directive laws, living wills and durable powers of attorney are still technically available and have been used.

Unfortunately, living wills might affect the likelihood that you will be able to survive a life-threatening illness in that many state living will laws establish harsh sanctions for physicians who fail to allow a patient to die while giving broad protection to those who allow a patient to die. This makes it difficult in borderline cases. If the physician does attempt to extend your life, he or she could be liable for the pain, suffering, and medical expenses that result from that extra life. Durable powers of attorney avoid this problem.

State living will laws, such as the one in Ohio, tend to emphasize the reduction of care for those who want to hasten death and de-emphasize the use of advance directives to make a legal statement that you would like to receive aggressive care. The American Life League of Stafford, Virginia, a pro-life group, has released what it calls a "loving will" that expresses an anti-euthanasia position. This document rejects the idea that food and water are extraordinary medical treatments.

Classifying the withholding of food and water the same as removing a respirator presents a problem. Withholding a respirator expresses hope the person can live without extraordinary means. Withholding food and water leaves no hope. A genuine "slippery slope" ethical argument develops that says this practice will lead to the next step of legally sanctioned, active euthanasia. It generally takes patients more than a week to die after withholding food and water, which puts a strain on the caregivers. Since death is assured anyway, the impetus for just giving the patient an overdose of drugs becomes almost overpowering.

Euthanasia-related Ethical Issues

Euthanasia poses numerous ethically charged questions in its own right, but is also directly or indirectly related to certain other ethical dilemmas, requiring even more complex questions to be answered, such as those below.

Definition of death. Euthanasia means an easy death, but what is death? How can we know when a person has died—the end of a heartbeat, the end of all brain waves, the end of interpersonal communication, the necrosis of the brain tissue?

Organ transplantation. When can life-sustaining organs be taken from a patient, and should the doctor who is planning to "pull the plug" on the donor's respirator be the doctor of the patient who needs the organ to live (conflict of interest and definition of death dilemmas)?

Abortion and the beginning of life. Is it ethical to abort an unborn child for the child's own good—a "mercy killing" abortion as opposed to an abortion done for the mother's desire or benefit? Should so-called "defective" children be allowed to be born alive? Should such a child be allowed to sue his or her doctors (a "wrongful life" suit, which has been permitted in some jurisdictions) if the doctors did not counsel the child's mother about the desirability of aborting him or her? When does the individual life have moral standing? When can it be the subject of a possible mercy killing or homicide—at conception, at birth, at three years of age? Is it immoral for a woman to destroy her embryonic offspring by using an inter-uterine device (IUD) if she feels the offspring would be unhappy if born?

Health care costs. Should society pay for indigent people who want expensive extraordinary care, or should that care be allowed only to those who can afford to pay without government help? Should the elderly be denied expensive health care services, other than those which are palliative, once they reach a certain age (as recommended by Daniel Callahan)?[4]

Patient autonomy. When should a patient have a right to refuse care, and when should society have a right to demand that a patient remain alive? In the vast majority of cases a patient can refuse any type of care, though courts have limited this right in the case of routine care refused by someone who had minor dependents—such as a Jehovah's Witness refusing a blood transfusion and having several minor children. Can/should a person express autonomy by choosing euthanasia?

The quality of life versus the sanctity of life. Do various humans at various points in their lives have different moral worth? Does physical suffering mean a person has more right to end his or her life than someone with mental suffering or no suffering? Is life and its continuance always a sacred gift from God, or do lives have relative values of moral worth? Is the life of a terminally ill old man of less moral worth than the life of a healthy newborn baby?

To address these many questions would take several tomes, but in a sense the question of euthanasia comes down to a general principle: The active taking of human life or the refusing of non-extraordinary care is generally considered more ethically suspect than the voluntary refusal to undergo extraordinary and painful treatments. In between are the majority of issues, grayer areas with no popular or professional consensus.

The goal for society, and for each of us as decision-makers, should be to not die well in the health sense of the word "well," not hasten our lives while they are still truly lives. But this brings us back to the "quality of life" types of dilemmas, for if we believe that a life can have less value when suffering is present and/or when life is short, then we could be dying "ill" even when we decide to commit suicide in order to avoid even minor discomfort. In the final analysis, we each have a personal ability (but not an obligation) to decide whether or not we consider our own personal lives to have reached the point where we, from a subjective standpoint, feel we are no longer "well" enough to justify seeking care or even seeking food and water. To overstate the case, if because we did not get to see our favorite TV show we decide to starve ourselves to death, should society force-feed us? Most of us would say yes, but this consensus might disappear if we ask whether or not a severely handicapped Elizabeth Bovier[5] or a permanently comatose (but not "brain dead") Karen Quinlan[6], to mention two celebrated cases in the biomedical ethics literature, should be force-fed by society for years.

The question of euthanasia can be addressed on a societal policy level, or on a personal, what-I-want-for-me basis. Both levels raise issues of what are our personal moral responsibilities. On the issue of what society should do about euthanasia, particularly because of the efforts in California and Washington state to pass referenda to permit active voluntary, physician-administered euthanasia, it might be instructive to look at the only Western society of this century, other than the current court-sanctioned situation in the Netherlands, where active euthanasia was a national policy.

Case Study in Active Euthanasia Policy: Dr. Karl Brandt

The only public official in recent times who has administered an active euthanasia program for a country was Dr. Karl Brandt, Hitler's chief health official.[7] Brandt was not some Nazi neanderthal who went around machine-gunning sick people. He was a compassionate, expert medical professional trained in the scientifically respected German medical school system.

In the spring of 1939 Brandt had been asked by Hitler to look into a request made by the father of a deformed and apparently retarded child. Brandt recommended approval of the child's father's request to have the child destroyed. Brandt even said this was not an unusual decision for maternity wards in German hospitals.

Later, in 1939, Hitler told Brandt to initiate a secret euthanasia program aimed at deformed children and the incurably insane. The program was carried out with great efficiency, and tens of thousands of mental patients were given "deliverance" from life, but only after passing through a variety of tests and evaluations conducted by university professors and expert practitioners who at any point could remove a patient from the lists. The program's scope demanded new medical technologies for providing this deliverance, and soon led to an invention that proved very efficient: the first gas chamber. This technology was later adapted and expanded to accommodate more than one person at a time by SS Chief Himmler in the concentration camps.

The patients to be destroyed were generally not aware of their impending fate. Except for parents of deformed children, family members also were not asked for input because they were not considered able to make such judgments. Fake death certificates were produced and sent to the families of the mental patients that were killed. Jews, blacks, and gypsies in disproportionate numbers were reviewed for the program.

Euthanasia of deformed children continued until the end of the war, but euthanasia of the mentally ill ended in 1941, primarily because of opposition of German church leaders.

After the war, Brandt was charged at the Nuremberg trials with having committed crimes against humanity for his involvement in the euthanasia program and also for his failing to stop concentration camp medical experiments. He made an impassioned statement about the need to have pity on the incurable. Nevertheless, he was executed in February 1948.

My point is not that euthanasia is a Nazi philosophy, and that therefore all euthanasia must be evil by definition. However, one lesson from this is that when death is seen as a treatment, then medicine will allocate more and more resources to develop the technological advances to improve this treatment. Another lesson is that euthanasia has posed many difficult questions for many societies over many decades, and will do so more in the future, requiring constant vigilance.

The question of what to do to address these social-policy questions can be derived by appealing to society's basic value system. Unfortunately, in the 1990s there is no uniform value system, making social consensus difficult to obtain. This brings a situation where the law may increasingly permit or even encourage acts that a sizable group of Americans may find reprehensible. Even those who personally would consider such and such act a mortal sin might be willing to allow society to permit such acts for those of differing opinions. Then again, when basic values such as the nature and worth of human life are at issue, those who have, say, a sanctity of life viewpoint are unlikely to find it acceptable to avert their eyes from social policies that endorse the destruction or the abandonment of the innocent. The question for the morally strict to ask the morally lenient in these social debates is the following: "Although you disagree with my value system, do not you agree that I must strongly oppose you if I truly come to a personal ethical conclusion that your position is tantamount to killing innocent people? Would you really commend me if I were to remain silent at such a time?"

This argument is more biologically and ethically simple in the case of such still knotty issues as abortion, but is particularly complex in the matter of euthanasia. Euthanasia, in the author's opinion, is a more difficult issue on which to reach a black and white decision than is abortion. Euthanasia's most common and difficult dimensions are encountered not when there are confusions about the morality of taking the life of another entity, but rather when a living person voluntarily decides he or she no longer wishes to live.

If one decides one wants no further medical care other than palliative care, it is difficult for another person to say that further care is mandatory. Also, while I personally feel even less comfortable with the idea of someone having a "Dr. Death" actively assist him or her in self-destruction, it is a fine line, I admit, between allowing you to refuse to save your remaining life and allowing you to destroy that remaining life. And I do admit you have the right not to seek care in virtually all cases—even though I would not do the same. A national policy to restrict active euthanasia would seem moral and proper; a national policy to prohibit someone from refusing medical care would not.

A Personal View of How to Die Well

Here I pass from the philosophical and national policy positions we might wish to champion and move into a framework of personal communication. For those of us who share the values of Christianity and who seek God's pleasure, I would like to present my personal feelings about a Christian view of death—a view I present for the reader's consideration, not as a legal requirement for society, but as a possible course of action you might find helpful when you are facing your own death. This discussion will necessarily also conclude a personal view of euthanasia's likely benefit or disbenefit for me.

One of my most frequent prayers is for God to help me to "die well." By this I mean I want to come to my death acting in a way that God would consider "well done." I have given this no little amount of thought, and have reviewed the literature concerning the many complex burdens that death presents to us as mortal flesh. I have drawn some personal conclusions I wish to share with you in hope that they might be of comfort and practical use.

I am not terminally ill at the time I am writing this; if I were, my current calm and objective feelings about dying well might be difficult to maintain. From living on this earth for forty-eight years, forty of which have been as a Christian, I know that my moral maturity alters over time, and that what I advocate for myself and others at this time could well change before I come to my own death. Still, I have only the present in which to offer some well-meant advice that I believe is grounded in the Bible.

The basic question is how can we Christians forearm ourselves for a positive, life-affirming, God-affirming death? What lessons and wisdom can I personally find to prepare me for what may be the greatest emotional challenge of my life? Surely, there is comfort in the Christian life for those facing death. Surely God has given us scriptural advice and spiritual support systems that will meet our needs through our faith.

I desire to eventually see death not just as a grisly challenge with which, by the grace of God, I can cope, but as something to be in some way genuinely appreciated.

To appreciate death is a difficult task, for it is not something that persons find pleasant when it is encountered. Some who study the dying say that they go through certain psychological stages and encounter certain whole categories of common problems. The most well-known list is that made famous by the writings of Elisabeth Kubler-Ross: denial and isolation, anger, bargaining, depression, and acceptance.[8] Others, including Edwin Shneidman,[9] argue forcefully that there is no set sequence for the problems of dying and that each person dies in a unique way that mirrors their lives: facing the trials of death in much the same ways as they faced other major stress events during their lives.

Shneidman also expands the list of possible reactions to death to include more components than does Kubler-Ross; namely, "stoicism, rage, guilt, terror, cringing, fear, surrender, heroism, dependency, ennui, need for control, fight for autonomy and dignity, and denial."[10]

The Scriptures too often speak of death in unflattering tones. It is associated with the most grievous types of sins (a "sin worthy of death," Deut. 21:22) and with sin in general ("the wages of sin is death," Rom. 6:23). It is associated with sadness ("the sorrows of death compassed me," Ps. 18:4), and it is associated with fear ("the terrors of death are fallen upon me," Ps. 55:4). Death is characterized as being "bitter" (Eccl. 7:26), and as being the last "enemy" to be destroyed (1 Cor. 15:26).

However, the Scriptures also speak of the martyrs that faced death's terrors with great courage, from Old Testament heroes such as Shadrach, Meshach, and Abednego (Dan. 3) to New Testament heroes such as Stephen (Acts 7).

In the important example of how Jesus faced death, it is important to recognize that He knew with total certainty the type of humiliation, pain, and death that faced Him (John 18:4). He spoke of His coming death many times throughout His ministry (e.g., Mark 8:31), but it was in the twenty-four hours before He was to die that He seemed to face tremendous anguish over its coming. We see the loneliness of His impending death in the poignant passages about Jesus in the Garden of Gethsemane (Matt. 26). Here our Lord asks for the three disciples to remain awake with Him, but they fall asleep. Jesus prays that God will, if it is possible, let the cup pass from Him, but the cup remains. Then all the disciples abandon Him as He is arrested, tried, and executed. On the cross He cries out the prophetic words of the psalmist (Ps. 22:1): "My God, my God, why hast thou forsaken me?" (Mark 15:34).

But Jesus' historical message to us and His earthly words to us did not end with His death! The message the resurrected Jesus brought to His followers was a message of triumph over death itself—by His bodily presence back among the living. He returned to the disciples with a salutation of peace as they cowered together in a closed room (John 20:19), He walked with them on the road to Emmaus (Luke 24:13-35), He spoke to them of His eternal presence with them (Matt. 28:20). As Jesus had said about Himself, He was literally "the Life" (John 14:6).

The writer of Hebrews expresses Jesus' accomplishments in this way:

> But we see Jesus, who was made a little lower than the angels for the suffering of death, crowned with glory and honor; that he by the grace of God should taste death for every man. For it became him, for whom are all things, and by whom are all things, in bringing many sons unto glory, to make the captain of their salvation perfect through sufferings.... Forasmuch then as the children are partakers of flesh and blood, he also himself likewise took part of the same; that through death he might destroy him that had the power of death, that is, the devil; And deliver them who through fear of death were all their lifetime subject to bondage (Heb. 2:9-10, 14-15).

It seems to me it is the loneliness of death, or what Kubler-Ross refers to as isolation, that presents one of death's greatest challenges. We see the loneliness of Jesus as the disciples fall asleep, and we can feel the pain of the dying patient Kubler-Ross writes about who would take the hospital phone off the hook just to hear another human voice.[11]

Margaret and Lawrence Hyde have spoken of this death dilemma as follows:

> ...when patients reach terminal illness, they seem to know intuitively that they are going to die, and their mortality becomes very real. The greatest threat may then be fear of progressive isolation, the development of a sense of being alone.[12]

In the final analysis, we all face death singularly. It is a very personal event, even if we are with others who are also dying at the same time. The loss of our mortal existence, the cessation of the frame of life to which we are accustomed, the severing of every earthly bond, whether to persons or things—these are not losses to be viewed as minor. Yes, it can be comforting to be attended by friends and loved ones, and can be helpful to talk with others facing similar fates, but it is our own individual story that passes in front of our eyes. It is a personal event that cannot be experienced jointly in the same way by those who surround us, even though they may be suffering more acutely than we are with the thought of our death.

In this loneliness we find a cessation of everything we are and everything we hold dear, unless we have faith in an existence that transcends our material existence—a portion of our lives that is more than our bodies, more than our temporary biological existence. This is the glorious message of the resurrection. We must understand ourselves as having a portion that is outside the laws of thermodynamics, outside the entropy and chaos to which all matter proceeds, outside of the reach of a physical death. If we believe with all our hearts that our personality, our character, our free will—the essence of what it means to be us—will continue, then what isolation we feel can become that of someone taking a journey to a new home, a change of location rather than an ending.

The good news is that thanks to Jesus' sacrifice we can face death with a confidence that death is not the end. Yes, we are isolated from earthly friends and things, but death does not threaten any ending of our relationship with the One who is most important to our daily lives and our daily regimen. He who has created us is still with us. True, we have not seen Him in the same way we have seen our spouse, our home, our friends; but our experience of Him has been real and will only increase once we have left our material sheaths. The more we have laid up treasures in heaven, the more our hearts will be directed toward this transition not with an aura of loneliness, but of anticipation (Luke 12:34). Insofar as our self-actuation has not been directed primarily at earthly things and people, no matter how dear and how surely selected by God for our enjoyment while here, the joys promised for the next life will be clearly greater. It is only by leaving the joys we know that we can obtain the permanent joys we see now only "through a glass darkly" (1 Cor. 13:12). It is by putting our lives on the line for Jesus, by trusting in His ransom of us from the death demanded by our sin, and dying to self and selfishness, that we can find eternal life and eternal pleasure. In the words of Jesus:

> He that loveth his life shall lose it; and he that hateth his lifein this world shall keep it unto life eternal" (John 12:25).

Of great comfort to the dying Christian is also the fact that God is not unaware of our mortal plight.

> Precious in the sight of the Lord is the death of his saints (Ps. 116:15).

> Are not two sparrows sold for a farthing? and one of them shall not fall on the ground without your Father.

> But the very hairs of your head are all numbered. Fear
> ye not therefore, ye are of more value than many spar-
> rows (Matt. 10:29-31).

Our circumstances and pain are not overlooked by God; they
are precious to Him, and this gives our suffering meaning beyond
our ability to really understand. We accept our physical mortality
not because we enjoy it or see the reason why it came to be, but
because we have faith that God is aware of it, He loves us more
than we love ourselves, and He allows it to take place—just as He
allowed us to do evil things on this earth and still made a clear
path for us to dwell with Him after death, without sorrow, for eternity. Jesus said just prior to His "sparrows" comment above:

> And fear not them which kill the body, but are not
> able to kill the soul: but rather fear him which is able to
> destroy both soul and body in hell (Matt. 10:28).

According to the Revelation given by Jesus to the apostle John:

> And I saw the dead, small and great, stand before
> God; and the books were opened: and another book was
> opened, which is the book of life: and the dead were
> judged out of those things which were written in the
> books, according to their works. And the sea gave up
> the dead which were in it; and death and hell delivered
> up the dead which were in them: and they were judged
> every man according to their works. And death and hell
> were cast into the lake of fire. This is the second death.
> And whosoever was not found written in the book of life
> was cast into the lake of fire (Rev. 20:12-15).

> And God shall wipe away all tears from their eyes;
> and there shall be no more death, neither sorrow, nor
> crying, neither shall there be any more pain: for the for-
> mer things are passed away (Rev. 21:4).

A Personal View of Euthanasia

Based on these facts, I personally believe that I will face death,
if I see it coming, say, by cancer, without seeking euthanasia, passive or active. I know that death, even with its loneliness and terrors, is not enough to separate me from the love of God (Rom. 8:38-
39). If I find myself without a mind, I doubt that it will worry me
(!); if I have even temporary or permanent lucidity as I approach
death, then I will be able to still reach out to God and man through
a ministry of prayer, even if totally bedridden. If my health-care
expenses exceed my resources and exceed the money that my family will or can pay, and if the government considers me to be too

expensive to care for, those are decisions they will have to make. As for me, I plan to live out my life as long as God gives me life and apply my earthly resources to this purpose, trusting Him not to ask me to bear more than I can (1 Cor. 10:13), and avoiding any offers of "release by death" that require active euthanasia, the withdrawing of ordinary care (food and water), or the refusing of any reasonable medical intervention.

And just what is a reasonable medical intervention to me? I feel it would be anything that would prolong my physical life for more than a day or two. As for pain control that might end my life a little sooner, or which might give me a less than complete consciousness in order to avoid great suffering, I would accept that, based on the verse, "Give strong drink unto him that is ready to perish, and wine unto those that be of heavy hearts" (Prov. 31:6).

Nevertheless, I cannot be like those in the Hemlock Society and the Society for the Right to Die who tend to equate a suffering life with a meaningless life. We are called upon as Christians to take up our cross each day (Luke 9:23), to share in the sufferings of Christ (2 Cor. 1:5). I cannot knowingly tell the author of life that I have given up on the life He has given me. I cannot follow the examples of the prophets Jonah (Jonah 4:3) or Elijah (1 Kings 19:4) and pray (unsuccessfully) for the Lord to kill me. I cannot fail to see that God has set before me a path that leads I know not where, but leads to a destination that will ultimately please us both, for He knows all, He has made me, and He loves me. If we are faithful in using our lives to yield fruit for Him, I believe He will give us responsibilities and power beyond our wildest dreams. Jesus gave us some inkling of the contrast between our current state and the state we would enjoy in the next life when He spoke in the nineteenth chapter of Luke about the nobleman who left his ten servants ten pounds while he went to a far county to receive a kingdom. When the nobleman returned, he asked for an accounting, and to the one who had gained ten-fold he gave authority over ten cities.

Roughly speaking, this seems like a promise of a billion-fold increase in responsibility and resources. If we are faithful, the Savior will provide us with generous attributes and circumstances that will never be taken from us by death again—the rest of eternity will be a growing experience with more responsibility and no sorrowful separation—what we receive will truly be ours.

> If ye have not been faithful in that which is another
> man's, who shall give you that which is your own?
> (Luke 16:12).

I hope to have borne fruit for the Lord and to receive more resources and authority, permanently, in His kingdom. My primary concern on earth is neither seeking an easy life nor an easy death, though I am truly thankful that He has promised us that whatever yoke He placed upon us will be easy (Matt. 11:30). If I see death coming, I will no doubt pray for that cup to be passed from me, to be delayed, to be reduced in severity—but at some point, unless Jesus returns first, death will nevertheless finally come to Gary Crum.

In my last moments of mental clarity, I will find myself in close quarters with the final enemy. At that point I expect to find comfort in the fact that God knows the meaning of my suffering, and that I will appreciate Jesus more than ever before—for His having voluntarily suffered this final enemy himself, on my (and your) behalf. He has ransomed us at great expense.

Until then I will cherish the life I have been given by God until my tasks, sufferings, and prayers are through and I too can say it is finished. And then I will pass on to the next stage with anticipation—entering through death's door looking forward to meeting my Savior face to face even more than I mourn leaving the kindest aspects of this sin-tainted world.

Endnotes

[1]Derek Humphry, *Final Exit: The Practicalities of Self-deliverance and Assisted Suicide for the Dying* (Eugene, Ore.: The Hemlock Society, 1991).

[2]Ibid., 20.

[3]Ibid., 14.

[4]Daniel Callahan, *What Kind of Life? The Limits of Medical Progress* (New York: Simon & Schuster, 1990).

[5]See Humphry, 60.

[6]See Robert Wennberg, *Terminal Choices: Euthanasia, Suicide, and the Right to Die* (Grand Rapids: William B. Eerdmans Publishing Co., 1989), 164.

[7]Gary Crum, "Nazi Bioethics and a Doctor's Defense," *HumanLife Review* (Summer, 1982), 8(3): 55-69. (This article was based on the author's review of the Nuremberg transcripts on file at the U.S. National Archives.)

[8]Elisabeth Kubler-Ross, *On Death and Dying* (New York: Macmillan Publishing Co., 1969).

[9]Edwin Shneidman, *Voices of Death* (New York: Harper & Row, 1980).

[10]Ibid., 111.

[11]Kubler-Ross, 40.

[12]Margaret Hyde, and L.E. Hyde. *Meeting Death* (New York: Walker and Co., 1989), 56.

The Impact
of Suffering on
End-of-Life Decisions

By David B. Biebel

By the year 2000, we should be able to dial the local branch of the Fast Exit Obitorium. If we get through—the lines may be quite busy—we'll hear the friendly, electronically generated voice of Dr. Death: "Sorry, can't come to the phone right now. But at the tone, leave your name, age, telephone number and the date and time you wish to die. If you are under age seventy, we will send the certificate to the Commission on Heroic Acts and deposit the appropriate compensation to an account of your choice, minus the cost of our services. Otherwise, payment is cash, in advance. No credit cards."

Farfetched? Dr. Death's business card reads: "Jack Kevorkian, M.D., Bioethics and Obitiatry. Special death counseling by appointment only." He intends to set up suicide centers nationwide.

Kevorkian's co-champion of suicide facilitation, Derek Humphry—a founder of the Hemlock Society—argues that "suicide centers are unnecessary because, with a simple change in the law through the Death with Dignity Act (DDA), help with death could happen quietly at home or at the hospital as a privately negotiated arrangement between doctor and patient. Additionally, there could never be enough suicide centers across America within easy distance of people sick and unable to travel."[1]

Notice—there's not a hint that suicide centers would be a bad thing, only that if the law could be changed, such institutions would be superfluous because physician-providers would finally be free to deliver whatever the consumer-patient should order, including death.

Each of these proponents of medicalized killing has his own agenda. The good news is, so far the Hemlock Society has failed to pass variations of the DDA, first in the state of Washington in 1991 and then in California in 1992. My expectation is that they will never give up until the DDA is law in at least one state, after which the rest of the fight will be in the courts.

The bad news is, Kevorkian has intensified his campaign. Dr. Death launched himself into the limelight in June 1990, when he allowed a woman he hardly knew—Janet Adkins—to demonstrate the deadliness of his "suicide machine." The former pathologist's tally of victims had reached fifteen before Michigan Governor John Engler signed a bill on February 25, 1993, moving up the effective date of a new law outlawing assisting suicide. The governor's action was prompted by the fact that in the first eighteen days of February alone, Kevorkian had assisted six suicides. This frenzy was forced, according to one of Kevorkian's lawyers, not by his client, but by people desperate for the good doctor's help before March 30, when the new law was originally scheduled to take effect.

In other words, Kevorkian shouldn't be blamed that people were flocking to Michigan to kill themselves with his assistance. The real culprit was the Michigan Legislature, which compelled his clients, desperate to escape their pain (or even their fear of pain) to advance their ETDs. For if they waited too long, their savior might be crucified by religious bigots before he could deliver them, his carbon monoxide canister disconnected forever.

Although several good secular arguments can be made against physician aid-in-dying, Kevorkian and Humphry both realize that the only substantial hindrance to the fulfillment of their dreams is an archaic insistence on the absolute sanctity of human life, still being foisted upon the public by a moral majority on its way to becoming a persecuted remnant.

For example, immediately following the inaugural voyage of his suicide ship, Kevorkian described "his device as 'humane, dignified and painless'—and his critics as 'brainwashed ethicists' or 'religious nuts.'"[2]

In a subsequent interview, Kevorkian was asked if he felt Christians were his main opponents. "All the religious people!" he replied. "Those theologians, operating out of things two thousand years old. They should be operating out of medical books, not the Bible. Who really knows the reason for life? They say life is sacred, but when you cut me, I bleed. When I die, I'm an animal carcass."[3]

In *Final Exit,* Humphry wrote, "If you consider God the master of your fate, then read no further."[4] During a live radio debate with euthanasia opponent Dr. Robin Bernhoft, Humphry admitted that what he really wants to do is overturn Judeo-Christian ethics.[5]

Both men have been equally critical of traditional medicine, built as it is upon the alliance of Judeo-Christian values and the Hippocratic Oath, whose adherents pledge, among other things, to "use treatment to help the sick according to my ability and judgment, but I will never use it to injure or wrong them. I will not give poison to anyone though asked to do so, nor will I suggest such a plan."

But Kevorkian and Humphry—like the original Dr. Death—are masters of semantic obfuscation, especially in terms of reversing the meaning of a key phrase, "to help," in the oath just quoted. For example, after the death of Janet Adkins, Kevorkian insisted that "he wanted only to help patients in distress." He also boasted, "I'm trying to knock the medical profession into accepting its responsibilities, and those responsibilities include assisting their patients with death."[6]

Humphry's version of this line: "The role of the physician is both to cure and to relieve suffering. When cure is no longer possible and the patient seeks relief through euthanasia, the help of physicians is most appropriate."[7]

Of *course* the help of physicians is most appropriate; that's what they're pledged to do. But helping, in the Hippocratic tradition, means healing, if possible, and supporting when attempts to heal have failed. Hippocrates was a radical precisely because, unlike his medical contemporaries, he and his disciples categorically refused to either kill their patients or to provide them with the poison to kill themselves.

As anthropologist Margaret Mead explained,

For the first time in our tradition there was a complete separation between killing and curing. Throughout the primitive world the doctor and the sorcerer tended to be the same person. He with the power to kill had the power to cure.... He who had the power to cure would necessarily also be able to kill.

With the Greeks, the distinction was made clear. One profession...was to be dedicated completely to life under all circumstances, regardless of rank, age, or intellect—the life of a slave, the life of the Emperor, the life of a foreign man, the life of a defective child...but society always is attempting to make the physician into a killer—to kill the defective child at birth, to leave the sleeping pills beside the bed of the cancer patient.

The first part of Humphry's statement—that the physician's role is to cure and to relieve suffering—sounds so axiomatic it's hard to critique it. In fact, most physicians might agree that this summarizes their motivation for entering medicine, since these are the two primary expressions of their attempts to help their patients.

But, as Nigel Cameron shows in *The New Medicine: Life and Death After Hippocrates,* the fundamental tenet of Hippocratic medicine was always to heal, motivated by an unexpressed, but very real, compassion.[9] Relief of suffering was a byproduct of this commitment to help.

Today, however, cure of disease and relief of suffering have become medicine's twin towers, the former driven by a mechanistic view of human beings and the latter driven by a poorly defined sense of compassion, with patient autonomy the guiding principle and financial concerns sulking in the shadows.

Many doctors, especially the younger ones, believe, as Derek Humphry explains:

Speaking for myself, I would tend to choose a doctor under age forty-five.... My observation of hundreds of doctors...is that younger physicians are less dogmatic and self-opinionated. They are more open to new ideas, and better versed in today's medical controversies, including law and ethics, than their elders."[10]

Picture this: the old guard standing around the bed of a dying patient they refuse to kill, singing "Tradition," while the loud guffaws of medicine's new wave of physicians nearly drown out the sound of Hippocrates fiddling on the roof.

The emancipation from Hippocratic tradition leads inevitably to a free-for-all (or more accurately, a free-fall) in medical ethics, as Nigel Cameron explains:

> Once freed from the Hippocratic obligation to confine his role to healing, the physician is fatally compromised. The idea that his freedom to take an open-ended view of his patient's interests can serve those interests better, since he is freed from a narrow obligation to heal and not to harm, is illusory. His freedom in fact exposes him to competing pressures from which the Hippocratic commitment preserved him. The more diverse the range of moral options, the more complex the decision he faces, the more unpredictable their outcome.... The tradition of healing and the sanctity of life is giving place to another, in which a malleable notion of respect does duty for sanctity, and healing itself is displaced by the 'relief of suffering' as the chief goal of the medical enterprise, all in the service of an undefined 'compassion.'... Suffering may best be relieved by acting or failing to act so as to bring about the death of the patient. Human life may be 'respected' by being deliberately brought to a close. These are the radically new options being taken up in contemporary medicine.[11]

As you probably know, on Tuesday, February 9, 1993, lawmakers in the Netherlands' lower house of Parliament voted 91-46 to guarantee physicians immunity from prosecution for euthanizing their patients—at the patient's request—if strict guidelines established by the Royal Dutch Medical Association (RDMA) are followed. To summarize the most important guidelines, candidates for voluntary euthanasia must be well-informed, competent patients with a lasting longing for death, who are experiencing their suffering as perpetual, unbearable and hopeless. But they need not be terminally ill.

Obviously, Margaret Mead's claim that society is always attempting to make the physician into a killer is true. But the question begging an answer is, "Why?" Unraveling this mystery involves history, philosophy, psychology, anthropology, ethics, and theology. But there is one place all of these factors intersect—suffering.

Judging by the radical solution offered by euthanasia advocates, one would think that suffering is increasing at an alarming rate. But, without doubt, physical suffering was far worse in the days before aspirin, ibuprofen, Tylenol, novocaine, ether, morphine, or Demerol. It's certainly more than a little ironic that in a day when hospice physicians have demonstrated that most physical suffering of the terminally ill can be controlled through properly administered medication, pressure is increasing for physicians to put patients out of their misery in the name of compassion, in order to end their suffering.

As philosopher Peter Kreeft explains in his symphony of wisdom, *Making Sense Out of Suffering,* "Modern man does not have an answer to the question of why. Our society is the first one that simply does not give us any answer to the problem of suffering except a thousand means of avoiding it."[12]

The ultimate avoidance of anything is its destruction, but it requires a certain leap of irrationality to justify the destruction of a human being to end his or her suffering. That is, unless you espouse a totally secular, materialistic view of reality, in which case Jane Fonda's famous response to why she had blown away her constantly miserable companion, "They shoot horses, don't they?" seems to make sense. But does it, really?

Dr. James S. Goodwin, challenged this in "Mercy Killing: Mercy for Whom?" He said:

> Killing old, sick, injured, or unwanted animals is common in our society; it's a major function of humane societies. And the reason nearly always given is that we are doing it for the animals' sakes, that we are relieving (or sometimes preventing) their misery. This reasoning bears closer examination.
>
> Why do we shoot horses? There is no reason to think they want us to.... We kill horses and other animals because they cannot tell us not to. Their inability to communicate is coupled with our ignorance of their inner experience; we do not know what they are thinking, what they want.... Another reason for killing horses is the relief of suffering, but, we must ask, whose suffering is being relieved? When someone states, 'I couldn't stand to see her suffer,' whose suffering is taking precedence: that of the suffering animal or that of the human owner suffering feelings of helplessness or inconvenience?
>
> There can be few agonies as great as witnessing the mental deterioration of a loved one. In many ways, the individual has died, but the mourning process cannot be resolved because he or she lives on. Add to this the

physical burdens of caregiving for a demented relative, and it should be very clear who is suffering.[13]

A still vivid illustration of this factor occurred in the much-publicized case of Nancy Cruzan, whose parents petitioned the courts to allow the gastrostomy tube sustaining her existence—in what some described as a persistent vegetative state—to be withdrawn so she would die.

Time magazine's cover story "Love and Let Die" declared:

The Cruzan petition not only marks the first time the [U.S. Supreme] court has grappled with the agonizing 'right to die' dilemma; it may well be the most wrenching medical case ever argued before the high bench. To begin with, Nancy is not dying. She could live 30 years just as she is. And since she is awake but unaware, most doctors agree that she is not suffering. But her parents are suffering, for it is they who live with her living death. They are so convinced Nancy would not have wanted to go on this way that they have asked the courts for authorization to remove her feeding tube and 'let her go.'[14]

After Nancy died, by dehydration and/or starvation, I suggested in an editorial entitled "Who Killed Nancy Cruzan?" that she had not simply died, but had been killed, inhumanely, by comparison to the way one would end the life of an injured pet.[15] As a result, I received no letters of support from the thousands of Christian physicians receiving the magazine I was then editing. But I did receive several strong critiques, and a letter from Joe Cruzan, Nancy's father.

"In my opinion," he said, "you are merely another misguided, ignorant hypocrite whose care and compassion for others goes no farther than the end of your pious nose."[16]

Obviously, it's not very popular these days to maintain that withholding food and water from a person in a persistent vegetative state is neither right nor humane. But if the intention of any action or inaction is to cause another person's death, it is manslaughter at the very least, regardless of how compassionately the perpetrators feel about what they've done or even the patient in question. And—I hesitate to say this—if we're going to hasten someone's dying, even if we see it as letting them succumb to an irreversible disease process, dispatching such patients directly seems far more humane than consigning them to a slow death, regardless of their state of consciousness.

But my own answer to the editorial's question is "us." We all contributed to her death because over the past few years we have stood by while certain whole classes of vulnerable human beings were devalued, despite the bold lessons of recent history. But sometimes it seems that today's generation would rather write history as they go, by whatever rules seem best at any given moment, since anything older than they are is irrelevant.

One thing I learned by tackling that subject, however, was that the moral high ground is occupied by the suffering loved ones of incompetent patients—and their doctors. But on what basis does the mere fact that someone is suffering exempt their decisions from review? The danger is that by adopting this perspective we will become far too subjective and inevitably surrender to suffering, itself, rather than to the God who can redeem even the most abject suffering for His good purposes.

Based on our personal experience of losing one son to a rare metabolic disease that causes brain damage, and then eight years later almost losing another son to the same disease, I believe it is nearly impossible for people immersed in pain beyond their darkest imagination to be objective in relation to life and death decisions. First, you are afraid the patient might die, then you're afraid they won't. In more vulnerable moments, you wish they would die, especially if their condition will never improve. But then you chastise yourself for such a thought, suck in the gut, and do the best you can.

It is precisely at this juncture that the decision-making process can be very different for one who is a believer, especially if there is good family and church support. Unfortunately, the "Lone Ranger" mentality—rampant in our culture, and in most of us as individuals—dictates that we often make decisions without consulting others. Perhaps we fear they may disagree, or criticize us for asking hard questions that demand answers, when they're so used to answering questions nobody's asking that they haven't stopped to think these things through.

Beyond that is an unwritten social contract that we should not diminish someone else's happiness by dragging them into our unhappiness. But the main reason we don't think of involving our church is that based on our experience to date, the church is the only army that shoots its wounded. When you're already stressed beyond limits, you can't afford to risk abandonment, so it seems more prudent not to bother asking for help.

Yet God designed the life of faith to be shared. He shares His life with us through the indwelling Spirit, and we are to share that life with one another. When we face end-of-life decisions—as we all will—we simply cannot depend on our instincts or insights, since they are undoubtedly clouded by the pain we are experiencing. Nor can we count on the law to help, since what is legal may not be right. Even our doctors—if they have a secular world view—are not dependable for good guidance, because standards of care change over time, and what is standard these days may actually be an affront to the true giver, sustainer, and taker of life, God.

We need wisdom, which God promises to those who ask in faith. But wisdom acquired by faith will seek the godly counsel of many advisors. As John F. Kilner wrote in *Life on the Line*:

> ...discernment is more than an individual matter; it is profoundly shaped by one's community. The significance of community resides not merely in the way people tend to be influenced by the values of those around them. It also (and perhaps more importantly) involves the fact that what one experiences as an unacceptable burden is greatly dependent on who is available to help shoulder it. A patient's bad decisions may be as much the result of the failure of the patient's community to love as they are the result of any moral shortcomings on the patient's part.... There are better and worse decisions, and the better ones are rarely reached alone.[17]

So, in contrast to the isolation that marks our age and exacerbates suffering, let's involve the church in helping people make end-of-life decisions. The shared wisdom will help them overcome long-term guilt or remorse. And short-range, their experience of suffering will diminish, even before it is resolved, because a caring community is helping to carry it.

I'm not suggesting that suffering is a good thing, something we should seek out or force others to endure so God can have the opportunity to work it all together for good. To live is to suffer. It's been part of the human condition since the curse, and is still the reason creation itself groans, longing to be released from its bondage to futility (see Rom. 8:18-25).

Thankfully, God has provided those made in His image a way to escape this bondage now, not by potassium chloride, but by faith. For when we embrace suffering—our own or someone else's—and present it, and ourselves, to God as living sacrifices, we are using what Peter Kreeft called "spiritual judo" against our real enemy, the evil one, who keeps unbelievers subject to himself through their fear of death (Heb. 2:15), of which their suffering is their most vivid reminder.

Jesus called Satan "a murderer from the beginning...a liar, and the father of lies" (John 8:44, NIV). Satan loves to help people commit suicide, especially spiritual suicide. In terms of believers, suffering is one of his main tools in this endeavor. But by giving our suffering to God by faith, asking Him to redeem it for His good purposes, we use the evil one's move against him. Engaging in this struggle, we identify with the sufferings of Christ, and as a result gain power through our weakness (2 Cor. 12:9) and come to know God more personally and intimately, surely not what the evil one had in mind (see Job 42:5; Phil. 3:10-14). Not only that, as a result of passing through the fire without being destroyed, we have a hope within us that others who are suffering—they're all around us—will be driven to ask us about (see 1 Pet. 3:15).

When this happens, Satan has achieved the exact opposite of his intention, because his greatest lie is that everything is meaningless and without purpose, especially suffering.

This delusion of Dr. Death must be confronted. But before we charge into the fray, it's best to recognize that this engagement is out-and-out spiritual warfare. Putting on the full armor of God, therefore, is absolutely essential if we are to have any chance of victory (see Eph. 6: 10-17).

Perhaps even more fundamental, however, is an honest evaluation of how God-centered our end-of-life ethics really are. To get started, try answering this question:

If you were suffering from an untreatable terminal illness, would you want your physician to:

1. Keep you as comfortable as possible until death came;
2. Provide instruction and a means to end your own life;
3. End your life, as painlessly as possible, when you are ready?

I believe that, until we, individually, make an absolute commitment to serve the God who is for life by preserving and protecting all human life, regardless how compromised—including our own lives—we will not be able to authentically or effectively resist the lies of one who tirelessly roams this world, seeking whom he may devour.

Endnotes

[1]Derek Humphry, *Final Exit* (New York: Dell Publishing, 1992), 150.

[2]Nancy Gibbs, "Dr. Death's Suicide Machine," *Time,* 18 June 1990, 69.

[3]Rolf Zettersten, "A visit with 'Dr. Death,'" *Focus on the Family,* Sept. 1990, 23.

[4]Humphry, *Final Exit,* 4.

[5]Dave Biebel and Elaine Haft, "Dueling Over Death," *Physician,* Vol. 5, No. 1, January/February 1993, 10.

[6]"The Doctor's Suicide Van," *Newsweek,* 18 June 1990, 46.

[7]Humphry, *Final Exit,* 138.

[8]Margaret Mead, from a personal communication to Maurice Levine, *Psychiatry and Ethics* (New York, 1972), quoted in *The New Medicine: Life and Death After Hippocrates,* by Nigel M. de S. Cameron, (Wheaton, Ill.: Crossway, 1991), unnumbered preface to the preface.

[9]Nigel M. de S. Cameron, *The New Medicine: Life and Death After Hippocrates* (Wheaton, Ill.: Crossway Books, 1991), 65-67.

[10]Humphry, *Final Exit,* 10.

[17]Nigel M. de S. Cameron, *The New Medicine: Life and Death After Hippocrates* (Wheaton, Ill.: Crossway Books, 1991), 131-132.

[12]Peter Kreeft, *Making Sense Out of Suffering* (Ann Arbor, Mich.: Servant Books, 1986), 12.

[13]James S. Goodwin, "Mercy Killing: Mercy for Whom?" *The Journal of the American Medical Association,* 16 Jan. 1991, Vol. 265, No. 3, 326.

[14]Nancy Gibbs, "Love and Let Die," *Time,* 19 March 1990, 62.

[15]David B. Biebel, "Who Killed Nancy Cruzan? *Physician,* Vol. 3, No. 2, March/April 1991, 6.

[16]Joseph Cruzan, "Letter to the Editor," *Physician,* Vol. 3, No. 4, July/Aug. 1991, 23.

[17]John F. Kilner, Life on the Line (Grand Rapids, Mich: Eerdmans, 1992), 148-149.

Bibliography

"Perspectives" (Vol. 1, No. 1), including "Why Doctors Should Not Kill," and "The Power, But Not the Right," articles reprinted from the Spring, 1993 *Journal of the Christian Medical and Dental Society*; P.O. Box 830689, Richardson, Texas 75083-0689. Tel. (214) 783-8384.

Medical ethics:

Cameron, Nigel M. de S. *The New Medicine: Life and Death After Hippocrates* (Crossway Books, 1991).

Hauerwas, Stanley. *Naming the Silences: God, Medicine, and the Problem of Suffering* (Wm. B. Eerdmans, 1990).

Kilner, John F. *Life on the Line* (Wm. B. Eerdmans, 1992).

Orr, Robert D., David L. Schiedermayer and David B. Biebel. *Life and Death Decisions* (NavPress, 1989).

Suffering:

Frankl, Viktor E. *Man's Search for Meaning* (Washington Square, 1984).

Kreeft, Peter. *Making Sense Out of Suffering* (Servant Books, 1986).

Lewis, C.S. *A Grief Observed* (Seabury Press, 1973).

The Problem of Pain, (Fontana, 1940).

Tournier, Paul. *Creative Suffering* (Harper and Row, 1982).

Books related to the subject by David B. Biebel:

How to Help a Heartbroken Friend (T. Nelson, 1993).

If God Is So Good, Why Do I Hurt So Bad? (NavPress, 1989).

Jonathan, You Left Too Soon. (T. Nelson, 1981). This book is available from the author at: 505 Baptist Road, Colorado Springs, Col., 80921.

The Hemlock Letters*

By Mark Coppenger

Dear Hemlock,

I've been watching your work with great interest, torn between two desires. I do so enjoy the spectacle of cancer, the way it torments those wretched humans. But I'm anxious to seal their destiny in my glorious playroom, where I can visit torments of my own design.

If I could know for sure that they would continue to ignore Jesus, then I could relax and enjoy the show. But I lost a soul once by savoring his earthly agony. Some revolting Christian got to him with all that bloody talk about the cross, and the next thing I knew, he was in God's suffocating grasp.

So I must come out in favor of quick and certain death. It settles their destiny and gives me endless pleasure in this realm.

I must share an amusing story. You remember that pathetic woman in Michigan, the one who cried out for help in September of '92. Our good friend Dr. K expedited her consignment to our world, and now she's ours. Well, I heard her crying out for relief just the other day. She said she'd prefer cancer on earth to what she had now. Makes me proud. Lets me know we're not slipping.

I confess my continual amazement at how those loathsome creatures will leap out into the eternal unknown with so little assurance of a happy landing. Don't they ever think of the grim possibilities?

I'm grateful, of course, for the embarrassment the church feels over the notion of hell. You hardly hear it preached today. May it always be so.

Let me remind you that our magic word contest is still on. For every time you inspire someone to say "hellfire and brimstone," thus demeaning those who mention hell, you get a point. As long as we can convince people that talk of hell is oafish and mean and that God is sugary, we can calm their well-grounded fears.

I understand that Misogynes has run up a lot of points on the West Coast and that Misanthropes is coming up fast in New York. But you're not out of the running yet. Winners will be announced at Mardi Gras.

Of course, I'm talking about the amateur's game. Anybody can get a nominal Christian or a talk show host to say "hellfire and brimstone" in a superior way.

You might want to enter one of the advanced competitions. The big boys work on theologians, persuading them of one form of universalism or another. Get one of those prima donnas to teach that God is too nice to send anyone to hell, that God holds evangelistic rallies after death, or that any serious attempt at religion is good enough for God, and you've corrupted a generation of preachers. Makes 'em real smooth and laid back. Evangelism drops through the floor. They figure, quite consistently, "Why bother?"

Score one theologian or prominent preacher and you get ten points toward the big prize, a weekend in Atlantic City.

While you're at it, do your best to convince people that they're good enough for heaven. We're enjoying enormous success in this regard according to the latest polls. Just to catch you up, let me mention the strong showing of our celebrity division. By placing hell-bound stars in a good light on telethons, benefits and the like, we're teaching people that adultery and other forms of decadence are okay. Reject Jesus, sing "We are the world," and you're home free. Or so they and their brainless followers think. Oh, and by the way, don't you just love the way they've romanticized lethal sodomy with those red lapel ribbons. I'm wearing one myself. It's so much fun to shift those research dollars away from Alzheimer's and Hodgkins.

There's so much to do. Don't lose sight of your goal—to get as many people as you can both dead and here. So get to it.

Insidiously yours,
Dissemblion

Dear Hemlock,

Last week, I touched on the expression "hellfire and brimstone." Let me expand on that theme, the strategic importance of language. It's our most important tool.

Argument is fine so far as it goes, but it runs an enormous risk. Once you start reasoning with a person, then sound reason might intervene and all would be lost. It's much better to jimmy the vocabulary before it gets to the level of argument.

I suppose the German expression *Ubermensch* is my all-time favorite. Those dupes really thought there was such a thing as a master race. It gave them license to do all sorts of wonderful things—genocide, human experimentation, eugenics, euthanasia. Before that term ran its course, millions were slaughtered.

Today, "homophobia" is my darling. Just think of it. Let someone object to rimming and fisting, and he's branded a defective. Puts him in the same camp with those suffering from agoraphobia, acrophobia, and claustrophobia; he needs psychiatric care.

How does such a wonderful twist of language stay alive? Thank the media. Without their help, where would we be? They keep these words going, validating them by frequent and non-ironic use.

I want you to focus in the days ahead on those terms germane to your project. "Death with dignity" is enjoying good currency. Promote it. Never mind that true dignity calls for courage, grace, and a servant spirit in the midst of suffering. Never mind that these euthanasiacs are spiritually vacant. I think you can make the term "dignity" stick.

Whatever happened to those guys who, knowing they only had a short time left, determined to milk life for all it was worth? They'd right wrongs, renew friendships, venture ministries, and drink in new experiences. They clung to life, talking about how precious the moments seemed. You saw them in movies and such.

Well, I, for one, don't miss them. I much prefer the modern hedonists who go running to Dr. K when their days are painful and numbered.

Back to language. Let me recommend selective use of the word "rights." Play it down in China. Deliciously murderous totalitarian governments need the freedom to crush their people like insects, and rights talk gets in their way.

America is different. In free societies, rights talk can be appropriated by the forces of decadence and selfishness. It's our trump card.

The word's not entirely ours. I know you've heard all this "right to life" blather. But our people are the undisputed masters of rights talk. It's served us so beautifully. It keeps the conversation off dangerous topics such as wholesomeness.

The worst thing we can have is talk of good and evil. They always win on those terms. So, as quick as you can, charge the advocates for good with repression, paint them as threats to rights and you win. That way, you can put your people in a class with Abraham Lincoln and Thomas Jefferson.

I don't want to get you all worked up, but let me give you a glimpse of what's next on our agenda. If we can push through the right to euthanize, we'll go to work on incest rights. Some even say we've got a shot at legalizing pederasty. Who's to deny Johnny's right to have sex with Uncle Bud if both consent? Don't you see the possibilities if freedom is your only value?

The word "autonomy" is very helpful. Use it to cover all sorts of cancerous perversity. I don't care how wicked the deed, you can lend it an air of respectability by defending it on grounds of autonomy.

It's funny to see the damned speak of their precious autonomy while their Creator stands above and about them with all His divine prerogatives. Everything they own, every breath they take, is from Him. They're accountable to Him. And yet all we hear is autonomy, autonomy, autonomy. They're going to think autonomy. I can't wait.

Both words are serving our purposes beautifully in the case of medicide. Keeps the debate off such disgusting topics as the image of God and the stewardship of days.

> Grotesquely yours,
> Dissemblion

Dear Hemlock,

Don't let your enthusiasm for human pain and suffering blind you to its dangers. I enjoy their agony as much as the next guy, but I've seen it go bad.

Remember that fellow in Arkansas who used to run a shady salvage business. Sure he went to church, but his heart wasn't in it. We had him pretty much where we wanted him. But then he had that awesome accident with the gasoline and was burned to the third degree. It was great fun to watch, as were the debriding, the transplants, the bedsores, the scarring, and the tears of torture.

I can still hear the sniggering from Malodor and Bellum. But I can also hear their gasp when he turned to God.

It makes me sick to see that fellow serving Yahweh with all his heart. Would that there had been no burns. You know what they say, "A moment of pleasure. A lifetime of regret." So don't get too keen on the rush you get from human agony. It can backfire, and you'll have to live with a nauseating little missionary, spouting all sorts of damaging drivel. I think they call it "testimony."

With a little experience, you should be able to spot those humans who'll collapse under suffering. They're the ones who think they were put on earth for happiness instead of growth. When the pleasure goes, bingo! They're ready to check out. Never mind that they still have opportunity for spiritual victory and usefulness. That's not their cup of tea.

And don't forget about the family and friends. They can reach spiritual heights in caring for those who suffer. In fact, to my eyes, they most resemble God when they minister to the terminally ill. It's not a pretty sight.

We can't have these folks ennobling themselves in this way, so press for suicide. Rob their relatives of this opportunity to grow through sacrificial service.

I swear, this can be infectious. You know the old joke about the fellow who attended a fistfight, and a hockey game broke out? Well, just as there are cultures of violence, there can be cultures of convenience, where personal comfort is precious, and difficult life is disposable. I don't mean to be smug, but I think we're in the ballpark in the good ole U.S. of A.

When you come upon dying comfort junkies, turn up the heat. And for hell's sake, keep them away from analgesics. God didn't play fair in providing those to man. How are we going to hurry suicide when those deliciously diseased creatures can turn to chemistry for relief?

Derek Humphry has just published our own chemical "wine list."—"Madame, may I recommend the pancuronium, the phenobarbital, the potassium cyanide? The bouquet is really quite lovely. Best savored with plastic bag over the head."

I tell you, Hemlock, I'd do this for free.

Noxiously yours,
Dissemblion

Dear Hemlock,

You may recall that I spoke of the strategic importance of corrupt theologians. Well, we also prize corrupt doctors. Just as students can be sheep before their teachers, patients can be sheep before their physicians. Let a physician start working for us, and our population can grow appreciably.

Dr. K is fine for starters, but our public relations office quite correctly points out his image problem. He looks like Dr. Death. The haircut's dated, the grin maniacal, the personality strange. Not our idea of a poster boy.

Why can't you find someone who looks like Joseph Fletcher? He had that grandfatherly aura, with that spritely bow tie. He pushed our wares, but did so with charm. Compared to him, Jack's a goof. But you work with what you've got.

Don't take any doctor for granted. They are gatekeepers for the drugs that serve our purposes. But until they ditch that annoying Hippocratic Oath, we'll have a tough time recruiting them for killing. We hope that, one day before long, we'll see the emergence of a class of "obiatrists," analogous to paramedics, paralegals and midwives. Operating outside the Hippocratic Oath, and fully licensed to administer poison, they'll send a lot of folks our way.

But don't give up on doctors. They can paper over moral cracks with clinical, techno-professional language.

Now I don't mean to single out doctors for praise. Every profession has its own way of excusing its evil. You know those self-congratulatory and easily corruptible expressions, "academic freedom," "artistic freedom," "the people's right to know," "national security." I just have a weakness for doctors because they have their hands on all those lovely poisons.

I've been hard on Dr. K but I do love his zeal. Reminds me of a dedicated pimp. He pushes his wares, leading fools to ruin. "Hey, fella. I know you're hurtin'. Come on in. We'll give you good relief. Won't cost much. Make you feel better." Pimping. Pimping for death.

If they only knew how they'd feel just moments after he had his way with them. Like I said before, the cancer lady's a hoot. I can hear her howling now.

Infernally yours,
Dissemblion

Dear Hemlock,

The Directorate of Peer Pressure has undertaken a joint study with the Ministry of Money. They've been meeting in private, but rumor has it that they've discovered a whole new technique for delivering the damned.

Here's how it works: Fan the flames of materialism and self-indulgence with advertising and conspicuous consumption. String people out on credit buying and torment them with fear of financial shortfall. Stimulate greed in the medical and legal professions, driving up medical costs. Encourage litigation, which generates superfluous lab work. In short, make health care prohibitive and money an obsession.

The rest comes easy. The patient will worry about the expense of his care. He'll think about little Johnny's college fund and feel guilty. After all, the boy might have to work in the dish room at State U. instead of dining in splendor in the frat house at Ivy Hall. It's enough to make life itself seem rude. How dare they continue to consume dollars when career advantages are on the line?

See how the pressure works? It's really quite wonderful. Materialism and ambition bear fruit, and we have another citizen in hell.

You remember that old song, "Will the Circle Be Unbroken?" Well, not if I can help it. We can drag the whole family into this. By communicating exasperation at prolonged illness and then enjoying the economic advantage of euthanasic savings, they too are corrupted. A family fit for hell. My kinda folks.

Of course, you can work this scam on the patriotic level too. Let them fix on the national impact of skyrocketing health care costs, and they might just give Dr. K a call. After all, we wouldn't want to put a strain on America.

The upshot of this would be a growing sense of a "duty to die." If we could ever insinuate that expression into the vocabulary, then we'd reap a harvest of broken souls. Well, one can dream, can't he?

Let me say a word about your choice of leisure activities. If I ever catch you watching the Special Olympics again, I'll have your hide. I heard you cackling with delight at their limitations. That's fine so far as it goes. But don't you realize that those events honor retarded persons? How will we ever euthanize them if the public gets all smarmy over them? The Nazis had it right. Wake up, son. Those shows are counterproductive.

Try reading a little Nietzsche in your spare time, say his *Genealogy of Morals* or *Beyond Good and Evil*. He'll put a fine edge on your mind.

Demonically yours,
Dissemblion

Dear Hemlock,

As you know, my favorite art form is graffiti. I just love to see things vandalized. In fact, I love the original Vandals, but that's another story.

I can't stand the sight of God's creation, His pretty setup, all ordered and fruitful. I can't stand Him either—so high and mighty, so holier-than-thou. Makes me sick.

Put those together, and you see why I'm anxious to trash humans. I don't care how run-down they get, they still bear His repulsive image. You can find traces of conscience, of determination, of reason, of love. It's like fingernails on the blackboard. Puts my teeth on edge.

I know it bothers Him to see His special creatures, humankind, battered and marred. And anything that grieves Him tickles me.

If we could just get those bleeding hearts to see humans the way they see unwanted cats, then we could have a field day. You know how it works. Tabby gets on your nerves or starts to fail. Take her to the "animal shelter" for lights out.

Do what you can to focus their thinking on the similarities with the animals, and maybe they'll forget the radical differences. Next thing you know, we can have a chain of "human shelters" where they're goners if no one claims them.

Destructively yours,
Dissemblion

Dear Hemlock,

Have you noticed how much fun humans have skiing? There's something about the slopes that invigorates them.

Well, I love the slopes too, the slippery slopes. It's awfully hard to engineer great wrongs in an afternoon, but you can at least put folks on the downhill slide. It may take them years to get there, but the slippage is fun in the meantime.

Just think of what's happened in television, movies, and popular music. Even I'm not used to that much success that quickly. Why it seems just yesterday that Clark Gable shocked the nation with, "Frankly, Scarlett, I don't give a damn." Today, that's kiddie show language. Our progress makes me dizzy. They're not showing snuff films on network prime time yet, but, hey, the decade is young.

I worry sometimes that perversion is spreading too fast. Kinda alarms folks. You might need to slow things down a bit, or there'll be a backlash. Show a little finesse.

I'm encouraged by the results from the euthanasiasts in Holland. I knew they couldn't keep it bottled up. Looks like they're having a party over there.

Americans can brag about the conditions at Vail, Steamboat, Breckenridge or Aspen. Personally, I like to "ski" Holland. The slopes are fast and clear there.

I trust that we'll have some good skiing in America before long.

Deceptively yours,
Dissemblion

Dear Hemlock,

Have you ever seen those Western movies where they circle the wagons? Well, that's what I want you to do for the terminally ill. Keep them surrounded with hell-bound people. Regulate what they read.

Derek Humphry is particularly helpful. It's ironic that we'll torture him throughout eternity, given the great assistance he's rendered us. Imagine the look on his face when he meets us. I love this work, don't you?

Do your best to squelch anything on euthanasia by Koop, Pellegrino, Schaeffer, or Eareckson-Tada. That last one is particularly dangerous. How are we going to persuade people that catastrophic illness robs life of meaning when this quadriplegic, bed-sored twit is jabbering about the grace of God and carrying on a ministry?

I warn you, Hemlock, these humans can hurt you when they're down. I'll never forget that paralytic up in Canada who decided he'd spend his days in intercessory prayer. I swear, he shut down about five percent of our projects in Ontario. Was I relieved when he died. Every day he lived, his prayers confounded the efforts of at least one of your colleagues.

Keep the dying out of hospices, away from Christians, free of edifying companionship, ignorant of Scripture, and oblivious to the comfort of the Holy Spirit. If you let some compassionate believer through, who knows but our subject might get saved, filled with the Holy Spirit, equipped for ministry, and fruitful even in their dying days. I wretch to consider it, but it's possible. And woe to you if you let it happen. At the very least, you'll do without MTV for a year.

Relentlessly yours,
Dissemblion

Dear Hemlock,

I fully accept the fact that we just won't get certain people. Once God saves them they stay saved. I've never been able to snatch one from Him. But that doesn't mean we can't hassle them while they're still on earth. A little payback can be quite satisfying.

Death to the damned is, of course, our priority, but if you have any time left, I'd like you to oppress some of his children. I have a special one in mind.

His books have done us great harm, as have his sermons. His influence has been enormous, as has his joy. But now that he's dying, depression is starting to nibble at his spirit. We must build on this.

I'd like for you to whisper the "good sport" theme in his ear. Make him keenly aware of his diminished capacities. Help him to see himself as a burden to others. Lead him to think that suicide would be gentlemanly, saving dollars and trouble. Heap some false guilt on him.

Of course, his suicide would horrify and shame his friends, but depression makes people stupid. He might forget the grief it would bring them. And he might forget the fact that he's still capable of spiritual warfare. If you could stop just one prayer, one intrusive petition, your efforts would compensate for a multitude of regrettable goodness.

I must go now. There's a reception at the photographic gallery. The Mapplethorpe collection opens this evening.

I won't be writing for a while. You know, I'm not omnipotent, so I must budget my time. Things seem to be progressing nicely in your area, so I've decided to shift my attention to religious liberty. There's so much to undermine, and so little time.

I know you'll do your duty.

Yours in darkness,
Dissemblion

*With apologies to C. S. Lewis.

PART IV
Crisis for the People of Life

Reflections on Science, Technology, and Faith

By Thomas R. Harris

An intellectual movement currently popular on many campuses is that of "deconstructionism"—freeing works from the crust of bias and prejudice which surrounds them and looking at the underlying truth. Thus, I think it is important to state my viewpoint, if not bias, regarding the issues which I shall discuss. As I am a lifelong Southern Baptist who will soon celebrate his fiftieth year as a formal member of that denomination, my interest in this subject stems from trying to synthesize two somewhat divergent views of life—scientist and Christian—and through the stimulus of teaching college students at the First Baptist Church of Nashville, Tennessee.

I am a career academician with degrees in engineering and medicine. I have worked the last fifteen years in research on the pulmonary vascular system, with a particular emphasis on the pathophysiology of the Adult Respiratory Distress Syndrome.[1,2] This is a disease with about 60 percent mortality. It is characterized by increased capillary permeability in the lung microvessels and leads to severe lung fluid imbalance and excess fluid accumulations in the lung—pulmonary edema—which can, in turn, result in complete respiratory failure. Patients with ARDS usually reside in medical or surgical intensive care units (MICU, SICU). I have been interested in the basic physiology of this disease and the development of useful technology to diagnose and treat it. I am a licensed physician, but do not practice medicine in any routine way. My day is concerned with research on animal models of disease, cultured cell systems, biomathematics, medical instrumentation and computing, and the administration of a large academic program which supervises work toward B.E., M.S. and Ph.D. degrees in biomedical engineering. We define this field as the application of modern physical and engineering science to the problems of medicine and biology. Its scope varies from mathematical theory to the design of practical devices to improve health care in many settings.

I wish to identify with a specific theological position which I will define as evangelical and relatively conservative. This is a viewpoint which I think is at the gravitational center of Southern Baptists historically and is in substantial agreement with orthodox Christians of other denominations. What are the roles of such a religious perspective in the world of bioethics? Specifically, what role should the people who hold these views be playing in the current efforts to develop and apply rigorous ethics in the world of biomedicine?

In Pursuit of a Relationship

There is work to be done at the philosophical core of the relationship between Christianity and science. The nature of the problem is well illustrated by the following quotation by William Provine, a historian of science:

> The implications of modern science, however, are clearly inconsistent with most religious traditions. No purposive principles exist in nature. Organic evolution has occurred by various combinations of random genetic drift, natural selection, Mendelian heredity and many other purposeless mechanisms.... Humans and other animals make choices frequently, but these are determined by the interaction of heredity and environment and are not the result of free will. No inherent moral or ethical laws exist, nor are there absolute guiding principles for human society. The universe cares nothing for us and we have no ultimate meaning in life.

> Show me a person who says that science and religion are compatible, and I will show you a person who (1) is an effective atheist, or (2) believes things demon-

strably unscientific, or (3) asserts the existence of entities or processes for which no shred of evidence exists.[3]

The author goes on to state that probably the only reason modern scientists pretend to believe in religion is to prevent political
repercussions which would result in cuts in the funding of scientific research. Provine does conclude with a "nevertheless" quite typical of such attacks on religion. He says that, nevertheless, this
view in no way prevents a "robust moral and ethical basis to society."

It should be pointed out that this provocative article generated
a blizzard of letters and criticisms from scientists holding very different views.[4] My own reaction was initially somewhat opposite to
that intended by the critic. My feeling was that if this view of the
human condition were inextricably linked to the method and products of science, then the scientific effort to which I had dedicated
my life was a hideous mistake and false in method and concept.
This seemed so because the critic's views of human nature were so
inconsistent with my own experience. Upon reflection, however, I
decided that we were indebted to Dr. Provine for concisely stating
the conclusions regarding the nature of mankind which flow from
a rejection of all revelation or religious experience. His statement
starkly sets forth the inevitable conclusions which such a view
implies.

However, it does seem that too little is said regarding this issue
in the evangelical tradition. I searched with some difficulty for
what could be called a "Christian Doctrine of Technology."
Fortunately, some writers have dealt with aspects of this subject.
Many of these answers are complex and deal with similarities
between the thought processes of science and theology[5] or the similarities between religious phenomena and the phenomena of molecular science.[6] However, much simpler formulations may be helpful. There are biblical, historical, and philosophical guides to the
development of a doctrine of science and technology.

A few key passages set the stage for improved understanding.
The first chapter of Genesis reveals God as the Creator of the natural universe. The Psalm 104:1-5 reveals this same God not as the
divine clockmaker who withdraws from interaction with creation,
but as a loving Father who oversees and is engaged with all creation:

> Bless the Lord, O my soul. O Lord my God, thou art
> very great; thou art clothed with honour and majesty.
> Who coverest thyself with light as with a garment: who
> stretchest out the heavens like a curtain: Who layeth

the beams of his chambers in the waters: who maketh
the clouds his chariot: who walketh upon the wings of
the wind: Who maketh his angels spirits; his ministers
a flaming fire: Who laid the foundations of the earth,
that it should not be removed for ever.

The first chapter of the Gospel of John provides the link
between the Creator and the Savior: "In the beginning was the
Word," and deals with the issue of rejection by those who have
failed to recognize and acknowledge Him "and the darkness comprehended it not." These and other passages lay the foundations
for the Christian doctrine of science and technology: Pure science
is worship in that it seeks to reveal the details of the creation and
perceive God's laws of the physical universe. Technology is simply
the application of this same knowledge to help those in need of the
everyday necessities of life, including health care. Its basis is the
Sermon on the Mount and related injunctions to serve others.

But of course such proof texts are meaningful only to the person of faith or perhaps to the earnest seeker of knowledge. They
are of little use as return fire for the withering criticism of which
my earlier quotation is but an example. Is there an answer within
science itself? If anyone should understand the philosophical foundations and implications of science, it should be the founders of
science—those pioneers of previous centuries who originated the
discoveries and methods which make modern science possible. Was
their work possible only after they had perceived that "we have no
ultimate meaning in life"? Smethurst[7] has reviewed the recorded
religious ideas of many of the scientific founders. In spite of some
conflicts with the church authorities of their day, Copernicus,
Galileo and Kepler were earnest Christians. Robert Boyle, the
chemist, wrote more on theology than about science. Newton's
tutor at Cambridge was a churchman and a mathematician.
Newton himself, the founder of mathematical physics and the
inventor of calculus, wrote extensively (though controversially) on
the Christian faith.

Many scientists of this era were also Anglican churchmen.
Faraday frequently filled the pulpit of his local church. In recent
times volumes have been filled by scientists willing to express
their faith.[8,9] My own experience has led me to know many scientists and engineers whose religious ideas are well grounded and,
though sometimes unconventional, on the whole tend toward the
orthodox in their views. Somehow the practice of science seems to
have an effect on scientists which is quite different from the effect
engendered by philosophical speculation about what ultimate

meaning might lie in the implications of scientific work. But the critic will claim that early pioneers were simply trying to avoid being burned as heretics, and modern scientists have their eye on government support! Never mind that theologians of the seventeenth century populated pyres and prisons much more frequently than did scientists.

It has also been charged that the opinions of scientists on religion are useless because, after all, they are not trained in philosophy, and therefore they are unqualified to judge the larger meaning of their work. While there are many efforts to deal with this issue, one of the most profound is that of C. S. Lewis[10] in the little book *Miracles,* which is, in fact, more of a philosophical discussion of naturalism and supernaturalism than it is a treatise on miracles. It is an apologetic for the coexistence of faith and science. Lewis was profoundly disturbed by certain trends in the philosophy of science. Some of his concerns presage those of bioethics in his volume *The Abolition of Man.*[11] In *Miracles,* Lewis points out that the pure naturalist who holds the view briefly outlined by Provine denies the existence of rational thought. There can be no real science without free will. Otherwise, all of scientific thought is simply the product of an irrational, random natural "system" which came from nowhere and is going nowhere, and therefore cannot be believed. Lewis demonstrates convincingly that rationality and moral judgements are, in fact, examples of the supernatural—God—working His way into the natural. He discusses these and many other points in laying a philosophical basis for the interrelationship of science and faith.

Thus, there is ample material for a Christian doctrine of science and technology. But what is my point? I fear that evangelical and conservative Christianity is not coming to grips with these issues, particularly within higher education. While science courses are available at Baptist colleges, few make an effort to produce professional scientists. Baptist colleges rarely teach engineering. Few maintain ties with a school of medicine. The evangelical and conservative tradition has busily founded new colleges, promoted others to universities and worked on many areas of higher education—but expended little effort to create an in-depth dialogue between faith and science/technology. Such commitment may be necessary if the challenges inherent in bioethics are to be met.

The Scope of Bioethics

The field of bioethics has become a significant arena for the interaction of moral theology and modern medicine. Early emphasis on ethical considerations in hospital decisions came from Catholic hospitals and institutions where some of the first bioethics committees were formed.[12] One of the first treatises on ethical issues in life support came in a papal letter from Pius XII.[13] A great deal of effort has gone into defining the field. While an elaborate definition of principles is possible, much of current theory[14] deals with applying the principles of autonomy, beneficence, and justice to ethical dilemmas in a medical setting. Autonomy has been defined as respecting the right of individuals to make their own choices. Beneficence deals with the necessity that medical decisions should benefit, or at least not hurt ("nonmalfeasance") the patient. Finally, the principle of justice requires that all be treated equally and fairly in medical decisions.

The specific concerns of bioethicists have centered on the following:

1. Issues related to the beginning and end of life (abortion, the right to die, euthanasia, support of severely handicapped newborns).

2. The nature of the physician-patient relationship, including the personhood of the patient and issues of confidentiality.

3. Ethical dilemmas in the allocation of health care resources. This issue ranges from broad social policies to specific decisions regarding who should be admitted to an intensive care unit in conditions of scarcity.

4. The ethics of research involving human and animal subjects.

5. The ethics of genetic manipulation.

While other subjects are sometimes included, a great deal of applied bioethics centers on these five areas of interest. As stated earlier, theologians had significant influence on the development of the field, especially at Georgetown University. Much current work has become case-oriented, and effort is expended to train students and medical personnel through the case method. This has led some theologians to criticize the degree to which the field may have been reduced to pat formulae rather than broad principles.[15] Others have welcomed secularization,[16] while noting that principles free of particular bias are necessary in our diverse culture.

The ICU as a Setting for Bioethical Decision-making

I would like to focus on a subset of the broader problem of bioethics—the bioethical environment of the ICU. These units are special areas where advanced technology, biomedical science and human illness of great acuity are concentrated. They are relatively new innovations in medicine and are sometimes criticized as overly expensive for the results they achieve. Typical ICU's are described below. Each has developed from a particular technology associated with an organ system, but general principles are shared among them. General goals are outlined as follows:

1. Medical Intensive Care Unit (MICU). The original goal of this unit was to provide close scrutiny of patients on artificial ventilators. This goal is still prominent, but patients may have a variety of organ system problems besides respiratory difficulty. Typical monitoring includes heart rate, electrocardiogram, systemic arterial blood pressure, body weight, arterial blood oxygenation, CO_2 and acid content ("blood gases"), measures of lung airway mechanics, overall fluid balance, medication history. In many cases, more invasive monitoring allows determination of total blood flow ("cardiac output") and pulmonary circuit pressures. Patients on ventilators require airway tubes ("intubation" or "tracheostomy"), and may be conscious or unconscious.

2. Coronary Care Unit (CCU). These units were devised in the 1960s to limit sudden death due to disturbances in the electrical activity of the heart ("cardiac arrhythmias"). Intensive monitoring of the electrocardiogram, frequently with computerized interpretation and classification of abnormal beats, is routine. The main business of this unit is to identify an arrhythmia and treat it with electroversion (electric shock) or medication. Physiologically unstable patients with coronary artery disease and myocardial infarctions (heart attacks) usually spend some time in this unit. Patients may also be monitored for variables discussed for the MICU.

3. Pediatric Intensive Care Unit (PICU). This unit operates in a manner similar to the MICU, but concentrates on pediatric patients.

4. Newborn Intensive Care Unit (NICU). This unit is dedicated to the problems of premature infants. A constellation of difficulties cluster about these very low birth weight patients. Small ventilators are frequently needed as prematurity is correlated with hyaline membrane disease of the lungs and respiratory failure. Infections and septic shock are seen, as well as difficulties accompanying premature liver function. The complexity of working with such small patients makes this a highly demanding unit for health care workers.

5. Surgical Intensive Care Unit (SICU). This unit is dedicated to post-surgical patients who may have respiratory or circulatory problems. Patients recovering from cardiothoracic procedures constitute a significant population. In many institutions severe trau-

ma patients will be housed in these units, although burns usually require more specialized facilities.

Bioethical Issues in the ICU

A number of the general issues of bioethics pertain to the situation in adult ICUs. Some of these issues have recently been discussed by Marsden.[17]

1. *Research and the ICU.* The effectiveness of ICUs depends on the body of scientific knowledge which has been and will be developed regarding the pathophysiology and therapeutics of patients under intensive care. This research generally stems from animal studies, usually of the cardiovascular and pulmonary systems. Animal research is necessary to provide vital data before candidate therapies are employed for clinical research or used in practice. Unless stringently justified, foregoing such investigation and instituting clinically an unproven therapy is unethical human experimentation. The ethics of animal research have been debated for many years. Yet, as pointed out by the National Academy of Sciences,[18] medical progress is virtually impossible without it. Cell cultures and mathematical models are useful but not sufficient for the development of new therapies. The ethical agent for review of this research is the animal experimentation committee which is mandated for all federally funded research institutions. Protocols are reviewed for protection against painful procedures, and all vertebrate animal research must be approved by this committee, which includes lay representation. Human studies are more complex. Scientific proof of the validity of a therapy—usually a medication—requires a double-blinded randomized study. This means that neither investigators nor subjects know whether they are receiving a placebo or an active agent. Results are masked until prearranged points in time to avoid bias.

"Randomized" refers to the necessity that patients not be selected by the investigators arbitrarily. All such studies require approval by a human experimentation committee. The committee reviews the details of an informed consent document in which the nature of the procedure, the risks and benefits of the treatment, and the potential value of the scientific results are disclosed to the potential subject and formal signed consent is obtained. Some ethical issues arise when an effective treatment begins to show significant patient improvement, yet the study is not complete. No one wants to be the last placebo-treated patient in an effective drug study. Therefore, prior arrangements are usually made for a monitoring committee which will review results at specified times and make the decision to halt the trial for one of two reasons: (1) the drug is very effective and withholding it from patients is unethical; (2) the drug is dangerous, and unexpected side effects not anticipated by animal research are apparent. Then the study is halted. Generally, neither of these cases are seen. Considerable integrity is required to maintain the protocol in the face of product champions who may not be viewing the results with sufficient objectivity. Another ethical issue arises in the ICU when an unconscious patient is appropriate for a study, but cannot give informed consent. Relatives are then asked to make the decision. This problem may require the review of a bioethics committee before a correct decision is possible.

2. *Allocation*. Ethical problems arise when a decision is necessary regarding the assignment of patients to ICU beds that are, at least temporarily, insufficient for demand. The ethical principles of beneficence and justice may collide when a patient might benefit from ICU care in the short term, but ultimately die of his or her current disease, whereas another patient would have a better chance for full recovery. A recent study has even shown that allocation of SICU beds in shortage situations was apparently dictated by hospital political prerogatives, not patient acuity.[19] These problems appear particularly vexing in health care systems based on socialized medicine rather than in the current U.S. system.[20] While technical improvements to decrease costs and the addition of more beds can alleviate this problem, bioethics committees may be called upon to help decide especially difficult cases. Improved methods for predicting disease outcome and the development of less expensive care alternatives are also important considerations.[21]

3. *Depersonalization*. The possibility that health care workers may tend to interact with their patients as objects, rather than as fellow human beings, has concerned many ethicists, theologians, and health care professionals.[22] The ICU, with its atmosphere of technology and specialized personnel, who may not have been involved with the patient prior to the acute exacerbation of the current illness, could be prone to this problem. There has been concern by nurses that they may degenerate into machine-tenders instead of patient care-givers. It is always necessary to maintain sensitivity to the welfare of patients, and the ICU does offer special difficulties. However, many of these can be addressed through visitation by supportive friends and relatives and good nursing care. In addition, improved technology can, in fact, free ICU nurs-

es from technical tasks to concentrate more fully on the care of the whole patient.

4. *Discontinuation of support.* The most demanding ethical questions in the ICU involve the discontinuation of support and the decision not to resuscitate certain hopelessly ill patients. The advent of cardiopulmonary support through powerful medication and artificial ventilation caused a redefinition of ancient concepts regarding death.[23] The cessation of circulation and breathing had historically constituted the definition of death, which may be considered "whole body death." In 1983, the President appointed a commission to study this issue. Their conclusions form the basis of current ethical and, to a large extent, legal practice in the U.S. This group defined death as whole brain death, in which both higher cortical functions and brain stem activity were no longer present.[24] Fairly precise criteria for electroencephalographic (EEG) evidence of deceased higher function were suggested. In addition, brain stem death was defined as absence of all reflexes and inability to breathe without artificial ventilation. This definition does not include persons in whom higher cortical functions are absent, but who retain brain stem function, exhibit reflexes, and can breath without aid. Such persons may be said to be dying or to be terminally ill, but not yet dead. A number of highly publicized legal cases involving the decision to terminate support for persons in this highly afflicted state have caused a considerable concern about the ethics of withdrawing support. This is an important problem involving autonomy of the patient (the right to die or the right to ordinary sustenance until death occurs), beneficence (to what degree are such patients benefitting from long-term support), and justice (to what extent do such hopeless patients have the right to use scarce critical care in lieu of a patient with a better chance of survival). Current practice has been outlined by Luce[25] and others.[26] The key feature has been the answer to the question: "What is the patient's will?" This becomes especially difficult when the patient is in an irreversible coma. Bioethics theory and current practice center on (1) the existence of a previous statement by the patient in a legal document or other statement regarding the situation for terminating care when medical judgement deems improvement impossible; (2) when no such statement exists, consultation with next of kin or legal agents regarding the best solution—this situation is usually referred to a bioethics committee for advice. However, recent court rulings have moved toward requiring a prior statement by the patient. In a recent study[27] of 274 patients dying in a hospital, about one-fourth of the 171 patients

who had do-not-resuscitate (DNR) orders had involved the patient in the decision. In other cases, the patients were not mentally competent (about half of the DNR patients) and had decisions made by family members in conjunction with physicians.

The ICUs present many difficult ethical questions, but recent recognition of this fact has led to the development of a body of ethical and legal code that addresses these issues. Reiser[28] recently summarized the issues of ethics in the ICUs in the following way:

> Intensive care is a symbol, a space, a technology, a clinical concept, an ethical imperative, a last resort. It attracts, it repels. It burdens, it helps. It bankrupts, it enriches. We would not give it up, but at times we wish we could. To some its machines sound a reassuring refrain; others hear it as a siren's song whose heartening meter will eventually become a dirge. The reaction of patients who are its labored agents, and of society who is its uneasy supporter betoken ambiguity: about selecting and removing patients from it, about the criteria of its success (discharge alive, length or quality of life after therapy), about its means and ends, its inputs and outcomes. Are they appropriate and proportional? All are matters to assess as the technology and presence of intensive care grows.

Some Final Observations

In many ways, the situation in bioethics appears to be well in hand: A body of theory and ethical knowledge exists; it has been codified into case histories which illustrate broad principles; much of the ethical basis has been enlightened by moral theology; working bioethics committees exist in many institutions; legal precedents have been established. Where, if anywhere, are the unaddressed problems?

For evangelical Christians, a problem exists in the discussion of fundamentals. To a large extent, evangelical and conservative Christianity has withdrawn from the science, technology, and Christianity discussion. Bioethics has a significant debt to Christian moral theology. However, this amounts to a savings account which cannot be continually drawn upon without renewal. Bioethics is not immune to the problems facing many aspects of American society. Current society has spent the reserves of moral insight and selfless dedication that in the past led people with spiritual insight to participate in the creation of our ethical institutions. There is evidence that many of our institutions are morally bankrupt. Evangelical and conservative Christianity has an obligation to become part of the discussion about the relevance of science and correct choices for the implementation of technology—to help rebuild these important reserves.

A second problem exists in the need for a specific effort in bioethics. Since competent, informed bioethics is of great importance to all, evangelical and conservative Christians need to ask themselves what we are doing to preserve and improve what we now have. It seems to me that this view of Christianity has been moving away from engagement with science, medicine and technology, not toward it. New institutions of higher learning have been founded by this wing of Christianity, but little serious effort has been expended in the direction of science. We are starting to leave these activities entirely up to the secular private and public institutions. Resources are always limited, but Catholic Christians can afford to maintain universities with respectable efforts in science, engineering, and medicine, whereas evangelicals seem to do little in the field. While costs are high, some effort in higher education in science, engineering, and medicine is not beyond the ability of the evangelical and conservative Christian community.

Another problem exists in the availability of people who have been trained in science and technology, and who have expressed the Christian faith. Effective bioethics requires more than books and theory. It requires people who are dedicated to trying to do the ethical thing and who recognize the intrinsic difficulties in the human soul which impel us in the opposite direction. Evangelical and conservative Christianity has the obligation to educate and train people with this view, and to influence institutions—even secular institutions—to practice these principles.

Finally, a significant problem exists in leaving science and technology to an ethics founded on nothing more than the "nevertheless" which Dr. Provine indicated was sufficient philosophical ground for pursuing a moral and ethical society. I am concerned that Dr. Provine's "nevertheless" is far too thin a shield to protect us from improper use of technology. A hardier faith is needed to maintain and improve our use of biomedical technology—to, in fact, protect us against the "abolition of man" which worried Lewis.

Endnotes

[1]T.R. Harris, G.R. Bernard, K.L. Brigham, S.B. Higgins, J.E. Rinaldo, H.S. Borovetz, W.J. Sibbald, K. Kariman, C.L. Sprung, "Lung microvascular transport properties measured by multiple

indicator dilution methods in ARDS patients: A comparison between patients reversing respiratory failure and those failing to reverse" (Am. Rev. Resp. Dis. 67, 1990): 280-292.

[2]T.R. Harris, R.J. Roselli, "The exchange of small molecules in the normal and abnormal lung circulatory bed," *Respiration Physiology: A Quantitative Approach*, Chang and Paiva, editors (New York: Dekker, 1989): 737-798.

[3]W. Provine, "Scientists, face it! Science and religion are incompatible," *The Scientist*, 2, No. 16, 1988, 10.

[4]Letters, *The Scientist* 2, No. 17, 1988, 12.

[5]L. Gilkey, "Theological frontiers: Implications for bioethics," 115-133, in *Theology and Bioethics*, E.E. Shelp, ed., Reidel, 1985.

[6]K. Heim, *Christian Faith and Natural Science* (New York: Harper, 1957).

[7]A.F. Smethurst, *Modern Science and Christian Belief* (Nashville: Abingdon, 1955).

[8]R.H. Bube, (ed) *The Encounter Between Christianity and Science* (Grand Rapids: Eerdmans, 1968).

[9]J.C. Monsma, (ed) *The Evidence of God in an Expanding Universe* (New York: Putnam's, 1958).

[10]C.S. Lewis, *Miracles: A Preliminary Study* (New York: Macmillan, 1978).

[11]C.S. Lewis, *The Abolition of Man* (New York: Macmillan, 1973).

[12]E.D. Pellegrino, J.P. Langan, J.C. Harvey, *Catholic Perspectives on Medical Morals* (Boston: Kluwer, 1989).

[13]S.J. Reiser, "The intensive care unit: The unfolding and ambiguities of survival therapy," *Int. J. of Tech. Assessment in Health Care*, 1992, 8: 382-394.

[14]J. Arras and N. Rhoden, *Ethical Issues in Modern Medicine*, (Mountain View: Mayfield, Calif., 1989).

[15]S. Hauerwas, "Salvation and health: Why medicine needs the church in Theology and Bioethics," E. Shelp, ed., (Boston, Reidel, 1985).

[16]H.T. Engelhardt, *The Foundations of Bioethics*, (New York: Oxford, 1986).

[17]C. Marsden, "An ethical assessment of intensive care." *Int. J. of Tech. Assessment in Health Care*, 1992, 8:408-418.

[18]K.J. Isselbacher, et al., *Science, Medicine, and Animals*, National Academy of Sciences, 1991.

[19]M.F. Marshall, K.J. Schwenzer, M. Orsina, J.C. Fletcher, C.G. Durbin, Jr., "Influence of political power, medical provincial-

ism, and economic incentives on the rationing of surgical intensive care unit beds," *Crit. Care Med.*, 1992, 20: 387-394.

[20]M. Rapin, "The ethics of intensive care," *Intensive Care Med.* 1987, 13:300-303.

[21]H.T. Englehart, "Medicine and the concept of person," 93-101, in *Contemporary Issues in Bioethics*, T.L. Beauchamp, and L. Walters, eds. (Belmont: Wadsworth, 1982).

[22]C. Marsden, "An ethical assessment of intensive care." *Int. J. of Tech. Assessment in Health Care*, 1992, 8:408-418.

[23]R.M. Veatch, "Whole brain, neocortical, and higher brain related concepts of death," 148-156 in Ethical Issues in Modern Medicine, J. Arras and N. Rhoden, eds., (Mountain View, Calif.: Mayfield, 1989).

[24]Excerpt from President's Commission for the Study of Ethical Problems in Medicine and Biomedical and Behavioral Research, 138-147 in *Ethical Issues in Modern Medicine*, J. Arras, and N. Rhoden, eds., (Mountain View, Calif.: Mayfield, 1989).

[25]J.M. Luce, "Ethical principles in intensive care," *J. Am. Med. Assoc.* 263, 1990: 696-700.

[26]T.A. Raffin, "Withholding and withdrawing life support," *Hospital Practice* (March 15, 1991): 133-155.

[27]K. Gleeson, and S. Wise, "The do-not-resuscitate order," *Ann. Int. Med.* 150: 1990: 1057-1060.

[28]S.J. Reiser, "The intensive care unit: The unfolding and ambiguities of survival therapy," *Int. J. of Tech. Assessment in Health Care*, 1992, 8: 382-394.

Living in God's Wrath

By John MacArthur

The cultural debate between Christianity and paganism is a broad subject, and there are many ways to approach it. My approach to any issue is going to be from the Bible because I am basically a Bible teacher, and that is the center and circumference of who I am and what I do. So, this chapter deals with what I believe to be the chaos of culture that we are experiencing as an ethical crisis.

One of the most tragic scenes on the pages of Scripture involves the strongest man who ever lived, a man named Samson, the original and only genuine Superman. In the Book of Judges we read the following account:

> When Delilah saw that he had told her everything, she sent word to the rulers of the Philistines, "Come back once more; he has told me everything." So the rulers of the Philistines returned with the silver in their hands. Having put him to sleep on her lap, she called a man to shave off the seven braids of his hair, and so began to subdue him. And his strength left him. Then she called, "Samson, the Philistines are upon you!" He awoke from his sleep and thought, "I'll go out as before and shake myself free." But he did not know that the Lord had left him. Then the Philistines seized him, gouged out his eyes and took him down to Gaza.

Binding him with bronze shackles, they set him to grinding in the prison (Judg. 16:18-21, NIV).

Samson did not know that the Lord had departed from him. It was not just a personal tragedy in the Old Testament. It was a national tragedy for the sons of Israel because in Judges 10:13-14 (KJV) God said, "Ye have forsaken me, and served other gods: wherefore I will deliver you no more. Go and cry unto the gods which ye have chosen; let them deliver you in the time of your tribulation." Proverbs 1:24-31 (NIV) expresses a very similar sentiment:

> But since you rejected me when I called and no one gave heed when I stretched out my hand, since you ignored all my advice and would not accept my rebuke, I in turn will laugh at your disaster; I will mock when calamity overtakes you—when calamity overtakes you like a storm, when disaster sweeps over you like a whirlwind, when distress and troubles overwhelm you. Then they will call to me but I will not answer; they will look for me but will not find me. Since they hated knowledge and did not choose to fear the Lord, since they would not accept my advice and spurned my rebuke, they will eat the fruit of their ways and be filled with the fruit of their schemes.

There are poignant words in Hosea 4:17 (NIV) where it is recorded that God said, "Ephraim is joined to idols; leave him alone!"

God comes to a point where He lets a nation go the way of its own choices, abandoned by God. You see it even in the New Testament, as Matthew records for us those devastating words out of the mouth of Jesus regarding the Pharisees and all who followed them and the leadership of Israel. Jesus said, "Let them alone: they be blind leaders of the blind" (Matt. 15:14, KJV).

I believe it is this kind of abandonment by God that we are experiencing in this country. I believe God has allowed this country to go the way of its own choices.

Paul said it this way: "In the past, he let all nations go their own way" (Acts 14:16, NIV). The history of the world is, in effect, the judgment of the world.

C. S. Lewis, writing in a similar vein in his book, *The Problem of Pain,* said: "[The lost] enjoy forever the horrible freedom they have demanded, and are therefore self-enslaved."[1] But there is no commentary on being abandoned by God that is as clear, as concise, and as penetrating as that recorded in Romans 1. It is the most graphic and comprehensive discussion of being abandoned by God anywhere, and it best explains the moral chaos and confusion that we are currently experiencing in our nation.

We are not on the brink of God's wrath in America. We are not anticipating God's wrath. We are not moving down a path to God's wrath. We are in it. We are experiencing it, not in its ultimate sense in terms of eternal punishment, not in its eschatological sense in terms of those events that will occur prior to the return of Christ. But in the sense of its temporal reality we are now experiencing the wrath of God.

> Therefore God gave them over in the sinful desires of their hearts to sexual impurity for the degrading of their bodies with one another. They exchanged the truth of God for a lie, and worshiped and served created things rather than the Creator—who is forever praised. Amen. Because of this, God gave them over to shameful lusts. Even their women exchanged natural relations for unnatural ones. In the same way the men also abandoned natural relations with women and were inflamed with lust for one another. Men committed indecent acts with other men, and received in themselves the due penalty for their perversion. Furthermore, since they did not think it worthwhile to retain the knowledge God, he gave them over to a depraved mind, to do what ought not to be done. They have become filled with every kind of wickedness, evil, greed and depravity. They are full of envy, murder, strife, deceit and malice. They are gossips, slanderers, God-haters, insolent, arrogant and boastful; they invent ways of doing evil; they disobey their parents; they are senseless, faithless, heartless, ruthless. Although they know God's righteous decree that those who do such things deserve death, they not only continue to do these very things but also approve of those who practice them (Rom. 1:24-32, NIV).

This familiar text holds a very apt analysis of what we are experiencing. In verse 24, verse 26, and verse 28, there is the use of the Greek verb, *paradidomi,* which is translated "God gave them over." That verb is used in the Greek language for the sentencing by a judge. Here you have the Judge of all the earth handing out a criminal sentence and turning the prisoner over to the executioner. Each use of the phrase in these verses expresses the fact that the wrath of God has acted judicially to sentence men.

God lets them go, not to eschatological wrath and not to ultimate and eternal wrath yet, but to the temporal and inevitable consequence of their own choices.

To put it another way, they are deprived of restraining grace. Sin is both the cause and the effect. It is both the reason and the result of their choices. Wrath, then, leads to more heinous and more blatant and more violent sin by virtue of the absence of God's restraining grace. There is definitely a progression here. First of all, it says in verse 24, "God gave them over in the sinful desires of their hearts," and He connects it with the word "impurity." In other words, they had no outside controlling factors. They were literally abandoned to the choices that their own desires generated. Man, abandoned by God, given over by God, sentenced by God, operates then out of the passions of his impure heart.

Jesus put it this way, "Nothing outside a man can make him 'unclean' by going into him. Rather, it is what comes out of a man that makes him 'unclean'" (Mark 7:15-16, NIV). The general character of people—the pornographic lusts of their own hearts that lead them to moral perversion and sexual perversion and to all other kinds of sins—are unrestrained. God just takes the wraps off. Of course, it doesn't stop there, obviously. Verse 24 says that what comes up from the inside results in the body's being dishonored. The scene is played out visibly in the physical form. The heart is wicked; the heart is unrestrained. The cultural props are knocked out that somehow suspend morality to some degree, and every person does literally what is right in his or her own eyes.

Alan Johnson writes, "In their freedom from God's absolutes, they turned to perversion and even inversion of the created order. In the end their humanism (man-centeredness) resulted in dehumanization."[2] And so the wretchedness of their unrestrained heart then gives license to the body, and the body runs wild in abuse and sex and alcohol and drugs and abortion and euthanasia, obviously propelled by a low view of everybody but themselves. Isn't it a conundrum of some sort that we have this massive enterprise developing self-esteem but it is all *self*-esteem and there is no esteem for anybody else?

Then in verse 26 the slide plunges even further. God has already given them over to the lusts of their hearts, which results in their bodies being dishonored among them, and that would probably speak of just the general kind of immorality that characterizes a culture. But now the slide goes deeper into the pit in verse 26 because God gives them over to degrading passions. That goes even further, and He names it: homosexuality. Women exchanging the natural function for that which is unnatural. Vile desires, gross affections, the degenerate and unrestrained heart takes the body and uses it as an instrument for degraded passion; and it goes to the pit of the unthinkable, namely, homosexuality. It is curious that the Holy Spirit uses women as the first illustration of this, because we all know that there are far fewer lesbians than there are homosexual men. The men greatly outnumber the women. Why does the Holy Spirit mention women first? Because in any culture, the last to be affected by the decay are the women. Instinctively, they are followers. Instinctively, they care about their children. They hold tightly to the values of the home, more tightly than the men. The point here of putting the women first is to show you and give you absolute proof that all virtue is gone. It has even invaded the distaff side.

The base inversion of God's created order then descends, of course, in verse 27, including the men who are engaged in homosexuality. At the end of the verse it says they "received in themselves the due penalty for their perversion." They get what they ask for. That's right. Built into the very warp and woof of iniquity is its own penalty, and God just steps back.

People ask me all the time, "Is AIDS the judgment of God?" Of course it is. But it isn't as if God is up there going, "Zap, you get AIDS." It is that AIDS is the product of perversion. It is built into the fabric of sin just like any other venereal disease. And so their own lives are destroyed morally, mentally, emotionally, physically, medically. Everything that seemed once so sweet becomes hopelessly bitter, and there is no mitigation of the consequences. But this isn't the bottom yet.

See verse 28: "And just as they did not see fit to acknowledge God any longer"—here we hit rock bottom—"God gave them over to a depraved mind." What does that mean? Sometimes it says "reprobate mind." It's a simple Greek word which means "tested and found useless." In other words it is something which was tested and disqualified for its intended use. It's a wheel that doesn't go around, a gear with no teeth, a spoon with a hole in it, a glass with no bottom. It's useless for its intended function. Unfortunately, those kinds of minds are running our country. The reasoning faculty is so corrupt that it must be rejected. It is not rational, not reasonable. The intellectual faculty does not function properly. The conscience is defiled because the whole creature is controlled by degraded passion.

It starts with a wicked heart, ends with a degraded body, winds up in perversion and inversion, and finally degenerates the mind so that it is useless. Then where does that lead? Verse 29 says they do things that are not right, all kinds of things that are unrighteous, wicked, greedy, and evil—envy, murder, strife, deceit, malice, gossip, slander, and so on. It's all there. That sounds like the stuff you read in the paper every day. Then, without conscience and without rationality, even though down deep inside they know the consequence for people who do the things they do, they not only do them, they give hearty approval to those who practice them. I can just see, in that last line, the studio audience on a popular daytime talk show applauding the perverts on the stage.

Without conscience, without fear, without reason, without understanding, and worst of all, without divine restraint, they reach the lowest point of human descent. This is where the abandonment by God leads. I read that, and I say, "That's where we are!" We are not waiting for the judgment of God; we are *in* it. The wrath of God is already at work in our society.

There is no surer token of a society under God's wrath than when it does not tolerate anger against sin.

The question comes, "Why would God abandon us? Why would He do this?" The answer comes back in Romans 1:18 (NIV): "The wrath of God is being revealed from heaven against all the godlessness and wickedness of men who suppress the truth." There's the problem. They had the truth, but they suppressed it.

I just read a new book by Wendy Kaminer, titled *I'm Dysfunctional, You're Dysfunctional*. This whole book is written to chronicle the fact that this country no longer accepts sin as any kind of definition of human behavior. The author suggests that the new anthropology/psychology/theology involves an utter denial of personal responsibility for any sin. She writes,

> No matter how bad you've been in the narcissistic 1970s and the acquisitive 1980s, no matter how many drugs you've ingested or sex acts performed, or how much corruption enjoyed, you're still essentially innocent: The divine child inside you is always untouched by the worst of your sins.[3]

> Inside every addict (that's the new term for sinner) is a holy child yearning to be free. Inner children are always good—innocent and pure—like the most sentimentalized Dickens characters, which means that people are essentially good and...evil is merely a dysfunction."[4]

219

The therapeutic view of evil as sickness, not sin, is strong in codependency theory. Shaming children is considered the primary form of abuse. Sickness is far more marketable than sin.

You may have heard of or read the book, *Diseasing of America,* where every kind of human behavior, no matter how deviated it might be by moral standards, is redefined in a medical or quasi-medical term.[5] Big business! And it puts the church out of business because we don't do medicine, we do spiritual ministry. If all human behavior is reclassified in other than spiritual terms, we are out of business.

We are experiencing the wrath of God because we not only have abandoned God first, but we have even denied the reality of sin. So Paul says in verse 18 the wrath of God is revealed from heaven against all ungodliness and unrighteousness of men who do what we have done. We have suppressed the truth every-where—in the Senate, and the House, and the courts, and the Executive branch, and the schools, and the states—everywhere. Somebody asks, "Why does a gracious, loving God, who is not will-ing that any should perish, but all should come to repentance, abandon us?" The answer is, "Because we abandoned Him!" Literally that verse says that God puts His wrath to work on those who suppress the truth in unrighteous conduct. Our culture has assaulted the divine standard, ignored it, rejected it, and tried to suppress it. God has said, "You made your choice. You are left to the consequence of it."

Four "Rs" Behind Wrath

Like all cultures which experience God's wrath, we have gone through the same four-fold process. There are four things revealed in this text that release the wrath of God. (1) *Revelation.* Men have been given the truth. See verse 19: "What may be known about God is plain to them." We have evidence of God in creation that makes us without excuse. God has inlaid into the very life of each of us the knowledge of ourself. He has inlaid the evidence of His existence and of moral truth in the very nature of our being. It is in our rationality, in our reason. So we are not without witness. In our mind is imbedded the obvious reality that for every effect there is a cause. It is also in our conscience, in which there is inlaid the fabric of a sense of what is right and what is wrong. It is as much a part of us as any other piece of the human anatomy or soul. We cannot plead ignorance apart from special revelation and say, "We didn't have the Bible. We didn't know." See Romans 2, verses 14 and 15. Pagans without the written Word still show evidence of the law written in their hearts. They can know the creation of God through their rational minds, and they can understand moral truth through their conscience and its facility to accuse or defend. John said, in John 1:9, that Christ is the light that lights every man who comes into the world.

Two illustrations provide samples of what I believe was and should be the continual pattern of evangelization regarding the gospel given to pagans. Acts 14 (NIV) shows how the apostles always evangelized pagans. Paul and Barnabas were ministering in Lystra and the people wanted to turn them into deities. In verse 15 they said, "Men, why are you doing this? We too are only men, human like you. We are bringing you good news, telling you to turn from these worthless things to the living God, who made heaven and earth and sea and everything in them." How do you evangelize a pagan? You start with creation. You start with an effect, because the natural mind is going to cry for a cause. The most devastating philosophy that has ever hit this country is evolution, because it cuts the legs out from under evangelization. If you don't need a cause for this effect, if you can explain the whole universe without God, you don't *need* God. But you are left with no starting point.

You remember Jonah, who took a short ride on a long fish. The pagans on the boat asked him, "What god do you worship?" He did not say, "Well, I'm an evangelical, orthodox, fundamental Jew." He didn't get into a lot of theological jargon. He said, "I worship the God who made the sea and the land." They could relate to that. They knew about the sea. They were surrounded by it. That was an effect that cried out for a cause.

On the other hand, whenever the apostles evangelized Jews, they started with Scripture. In Acts 17:23 Paul is up there on the hill with all the elite, the great minds of Athens. He says, "I was passing through, examining the objects of your worship, and I found an altar with the inscription, 'To an unknown god.' I would like to introduce you to him." Now he is talking to the elite, academia, the high-powered philosophers, but he doesn't go into some kind of esoteric philosophical discussion. He says, "He is the God who made everything." Just looking at God's creation is going to deliver you a tremendous amount of information about who He is. You're going to see that He is a God of order, a God of power, of beauty. You are going to see that He is a God of detail. He's a God of love, because the world shines in so many ways. Yet He's a God of severity, because there are so many tragic things. You can know so much about God just by reasoning from effect to cause—so much that if you don't believe in God you are absolutely without excuse.

Back in Romans 1, verse 20, Paul says the creation of the world was when it all started. Since the beginning of creation, God has always put Himself on display. His invisible attributes, His eternal power, His divine nature have been clearly seen and comprehended by human reason. You say, "Sure, we can understand that, but in ancient times they didn't have science like today. How much could they understand?" Don't underestimate ancient man. They could understand the fixed orders of the heavenly bodies. They could pick up a little flower and see the order and structure of the petals. They could see the cycle of water, the mystery of growth, of human birth, the glory of a sunrise, the heaving and crashing of the sea, the rush of the rivers, the flight of a bird, a caterpillar reborn as a butterfly, the joyful relationship of a mother and her baby—it's always been there. If there was ever a culture without excuse it is ours.

They now know that birds navigate by the stars. There's a fish called the archer fish that shoots insects with a stream of water out of his mouth—just for fun! Did you know that moths have a problem with mites getting in their ears? But you will never see more than one mite in a moth's ear, because if they get in both ears the moth will die. And how about those bombardier beetles? They squirt two kinds of poison to destroy their enemies, but somehow those two poisons never get mixed inside the beetle and destroy him. Ain't evolution grand!

You know what a massive operation it is to lift water out of the sea, put it in clouds, carry it over the land, and dump it? Every farmer in the state of Missouri every year gets half a million gallons of water dumped on his field in average rainfall per month and does not pay for it. What lifts that water? The sun, and it's 93 million miles away.

Robert Jastro, director of NASA's Goddard Institute for Space Studies, writes,

> Now we see how the astronomical evidence leads to a biblical view of the origin of the world. The details differ, but the essential elements in the astronomical and biblical accounts of Genesis are the same....
>
> Consider the enormity of the problem. Science has proven that the Universe exploded into being at a certain moment. It asks, What cause produced this effect? Who or what put the matter and energy into the Universe? Was the Universe created out of nothing, or

was it gathered together out of pre-existing materials? And science cannot answer these questions....

It seems as though science will never be able to raise the curtain on the mystery of creation. For the scientist who has lived by his faith in the power of reason, the story ends like a bad dream. He has scaled the mountains of ignorance; he is about to conquer the highest peak; as he pulls himself over the final rock, he is greeted by a band of theologians who have been sitting there for centuries.[6]

Any simple, primitive, or complex and sophisticated look at creation leads to the Creator.

Then you are going to have to ask the question, "How much eternal power does this Creator have?" Absolutely inconceivable power. Did you know that, at latest count, God made ten million kinds of insects? Did you know that the tail of a comet can be anywhere from ten thousand to a million miles long? In fact, some comets have a tail a hundred million miles long and move at 350 miles per second. How can anybody look at that and conclude there is no creator, no power source? But as one scientist admitted, "I reject the idea of a transcendent god, so what other options do I have?"

Men have experienced God, His wisdom, His power, His beauty, and His goodness in every moment of their existence, because it is in Him that they live and move and have their being. And as Acts 17:27 says, "He is never far from them."

Revelation is the first cause. Men have revelation. God has given it to them. They are without excuse.

The second cause: *rejection*. When they got the revelation, it says in verse 21, even though they knew God through their reason, they did not honor Him or give Him thanks for all the wondrous things He did. They became futile, or empty, in their thinking. After all God had done for them and revealed to them, they deliberately turned from the truth.

Donald Grey Barnhouse wrote:

Will God give man brains to see these things and will man then fail to exercise his will toward that God? The sorrowful answer is that both of these things are true. God will give a man brains to smelt iron and make a hammer head and nails. God will grow a tree and give man strength to cut it down and brains to fashion a hammer handle from its wood. And when man has the hammer and the nails, God will put out his hand and

let man drive nails through it and place Him on a cross
in the supreme demonstration that men are without
excuse.[7]

In today's world we see rejection in response to revelation. For all the joy, and all the beauty, and all the life and laughter and pain and tears, and all the thrills, and all the pleasure, and all the talent, and all the wonderful children and families and everything God gives, He gets no thanks, and no honor, and no respect, and no consideration. And He says, "I'm done. You go the way you have chosen. I leave you with your futile speculations, your empty human ideas."

God says to today's men and women, like to those in Isaiah's time, "You felt secure in your wickedness and said, 'No one sees me'" (Isa. 47:10, NASB). In other words, there is no one there. Your wisdom and knowledge have deluded you, for you have said in your heart, "I am, and there is no one else." This is the ultimate atheism.

As a result of that kind of rejection, their foolish hearts were darkened. You remove God, who is the light, and into the vacuum is sucked darkness. When God is gone you are left with intellectual darkness and moral darkness.

There's a third step in this process which led to God's abandonment. Let's call it *rationalization*. From revelation to rejection to rationalization, men insist they are doing fine. My own loose translation of Acts 17:22 goes like this: "Professing to be wise, really they are morons."

From my viewpoint, the major rationalization of our contemporary culture comes under one word: egalitarianism. It's the only morality we have—equal rights for everybody to do whatever they want. It's moronic, and it's reflective of the blackness that was sucked in by the vacuum when God was pushed out. I don't expect anything different from what I hear on Geraldo or Phil Donahue or coming out of Congress or from the news commentators. I don't expect to hear anything different from what I am hearing on college and university campuses, as professors of philosophy and ethics and sociology get up and espouse the blackness of their own souls, void of God. What is really kind of interesting is that they don't know they are moronic; they think they are wise—profound even.

Then the fourth, *religion*. They go from revelation to rejection to rationalization to religion. Men, having dispelled God, then create their own gods to accommodate their useless ideas. They have to bow somewhere. Voltaire once said "If God made us in His image we have certainly returned the compliment." In verse 23 it says they exchanged the glory of the incorruptible God for an image in the form of corruptible man and of birds and of four-footed animals and crawling creatures. In verse 25, they exchanged the truth of God for a lie; they worshiped and served the creature rather than the Creator. Again in verse 28, they did not like to retain God in their knowledge. So in place of the Creator they put the creation. They made their religion out of the creation. Maybe it was a figure carved out of wood or of stone or silver or gold. Certainly in animistic and polytheistic cultures it was like that. The gods we have made out of the creation today are a little different—whales, dolphins, spotted owls, eagles, "Mother Earth."

I'm teaching the Book of Revelation on Sunday nights, and the Book of Revelation is the environmentalists' worst nightmare. If they think we are messing up the earth, wait until they see what Jesus does to it. Man does not ascend from the muck of paganism to the height of religion. He falls from the truth of God to the muck of religion. That's the pit. Religion is not humankind at its highest, at its noblest. It is the ultimate insanity. It is the wickedness of mankind having reached its ultimate proportion—ridiculous, moronic, stupid. Having rejected the true God is one thing; having created a non-god compounds the idiocy. From the Roman eagle to the spotted owl, and the golden bulls of Egypt to the dolphins who have now been made equal citizens with the people in Malibu, from the worship of a stick to the worship of the earth, from the aboriginals to the environmentalists, from polytheism to pantheism, from Islam to eco-feminism, is it any wonder that our society is struggling with moral and ethical issues? We have rejected God, and God, in turn, has said, "America is joined to idols. Let them alone."

There is a species of ant in Africa that is huge! And they make anthills that are enormous, rising sometimes fifteen feet in the air. We are told that in these massive anthills, among millions of ants, there is one queen ant. Radiating from her are some kind of impulses like radar, and all these other ants obey her. The worker ants go out a long distance foraging for food and stuff to build the nest. They have to keep going further all the time because they strip whatever is near. They may go a long way out, but they never lose connection. Researchers who study those ants say that if the queen gets restless or disturbed, the workers, no matter how far away they are, become completely disoriented. And if the queen dies, they all commit suicide.

I look at our culture and I see this terrible disorientation. I see a new preoccupation with suicide. The king is not even dead, but they don't know it. Is there an answer? Psalm 81, verse 11 (NIV): "My people would not listen to me; Israel would not submit to me." And they are just a sample nation of what is going to happen to the rest—perhaps even faster, since we have no covenant with Him as a nation. So what did God do to Israel? Verse 12: "I gave them over." What did He give them over to? Eschatological judgment? No, that is yet to come. He just gave them over to "their stubborn hearts." You want it? You got it! He let them follow their own devices. In verse 13 we see the heart of God: "If my people would but listen to me, if Israel would follow my ways, how quickly would I subdue their enemies and turn my hand against their foes! Those who hate the Lord would cringe before him, and their punishment would last forever." Then in verse 16 He says, "You would be fed with the finest of wheat; with honey from the rock I would satisfy you." God is saying, "I took away my restraining grace, but I will send it back. I will give you the wheat and the honey, if you will just listen to my Word and walk in my way."

It has to start with the church. And we must call the nation to God, the Creator who is the gracious Redeemer.

Endnotes

[1]C.S. Lewis, *The Problem of Pain* (New York: MacMillan, 1962): 127-128.

[2]Alan F. Johnson, *Romans: The Freedom Letter,* Vol. 1 (Chicago: Moody, 1974): 35.

[3]Wendy Kaminer, *I'm Dysfunctional, You're Dysfunctional* (Reading, Mass.: Addison-Wesley, 1992): 20.

[4]Ibid., 18.

[5]Stanton Peele, *Diseasing of America* (Lexington, Mass.: Lexington, 1989).

[6]Robert Jastrow, *God and the Astronomers* (New York: W. W. Norton, 1978): 14, 114, 116.

[7]Donald Grey Barnhouse, *Man's Ruin, God's Wrath* (Grand Rapids: Eerdmans, 1952): 245.

The Sufficiency
of Scripture

By John MacArthur

When we consider the ethical or moral base upon which every decision is ultimately made, we find there are two bases, in fact. The first is general revelation, which is the revelation of God in creation. The second is special revelation, which is the revelation of God in Scripture.

Scripture becomes the second essential foundation for morality, for ethics, for decision-making, no matter how complex or difficult those decisions might be, no matter how far from any direct or immediate suggestion by Scripture they might be. Yet Scripture has to be the foundation upon which the initial thoughts are founded, the point of departure into whatever musings are necessitated by whatever difficulty the problem may bring.

The problem we face, however, is that our society has rejected general revelation. We saw that in Romans 1. Therefore, it has no commitment to a sovereign Creator. Willfully, our culture has rejected the rational revelation of cause and effect, and the truth that God can be known, and that all that is knowable about God, as Paul says, can be known about Him from creation and from reason, which is inlaid into the fabric of man's existence. We also noted that because the law of God is written in our hearts, we can know the essence of right and wrong. But once a person cuts himself off from a belief in God, he is then cut loose from any ethical and moral foundation. And the result is a damning kind of confusing condition that is even more intensified because, having cut himself off from God, he is then bereft of the revelation of God that is in the Scripture.

It is to that point I want to draw your attention. I want to teach the Bible; I don't want to deal in abstractions. So I invite your attention to a wonderful psalm, Psalm 19. The Word of God becomes the clarification and the codification of God's moral law. It is the only source of teaching about God that can save. General revelation gives us enough knowledge about God to damn us; special revelation gives us enough knowledge to save us. General revelation, then, must lead to special revelation. If you reject general revelation, there *is* no special revelation.

And so we want to establish not only the moral base on the nature of God as revealed to us in creation and reason, but we want to understand the moral base as revealed to us in Scripture. To do that, and not find ourselves wandering all over everywhere, I want to draw your attention to what I believe to be the most succinct and profound summary of Scripture in terms of its impact and effect on human life anywhere on the pages of Scripture—and that is in Psalm 19, verses 7-9. God, with that rather typical and amazing economy of words, says such immense profundity in such few statements.

Thomas Watson, the great Puritan, once wrote that the enemies of God have always been trying to blow out the candle of Scripture, but they have never been successful at it.[1] This is true. The Bible is inevitably attacked; it is attacked by those familiar people we call liberals. They just flatly deny its inerrancy, they deny its inspiration, they deny its divine authorship. We have dealt, I think, in some measure with that throughout the history of the church, and done so effectively. And then there is that more subtle and indirect attack on Scripture that comes from those who might be classified generally as existentialists. They don't necessarily overtly deny the Word; they would say that it does *contain* some kind of spiritual message which may be interpreted experientially, empirically, or mystically. God does speak in His Word, but they insist He does so existentially. Whatever happens to "zap" you becomes the Word of God. And then there are those who would say as well that the Bible does bring you into certain experiences by which God speaks—maybe revelations, words of knowledge, words of wisdom. And then there is what you might call a "primitivistic" approach to Scripture that says, "Well, the Bible is certainly a wonderful book spiritually, but it is naive in a scientifically advanced, sociologically advanced, and philosophically advanced, complex culture like ours. We would expect it to manifest primitive biases against things like homosexuality—its primitive nature does not comprehend the complexity and the advancement in human understanding."

Whatever it is, the Bible is inevitably being attacked. It is attacked blatantly and overtly. It is attacked subtly. It is somewhat patted on the head as if to be given some homage and not to be blamed for its ineptitude because of its antiquity. In all of those kinds of attacks, the Bible stands its ground. That last one bothers me. I wrote a book about this recently called *Our Sufficiency in Christ*,[2] and it is one of those themes I want to expand on a little bit in this psalm. It is this continual sort of harangue I hear about the Bible not quite being sufficient as a foundation for all spiritual and, therefore, moral and ethical issues. Even among people who would defend its inerrancy, and those who would defend its absolute divine authorship, there is being reflected today a concern, at least to me, that they don't believe in its sufficiency. Here are a couple of illustrations of that:

I was sitting in the living room of a pastor of a prominent church, and he said to me, "You know, I've just discovered tremendous new insights into leadership in the church." I said, "Really? Where did you find them?" And he named for me two new books written in the secular marketing field. One of them was written by a man who is well known for writing books on leadership; the other related to marketing and how to sell things to people. And I said, "You're telling me that these books have given you some new insight into how to lead the church? You mean the church of Jesus Christ, which He purchased with His own blood? You mean the church that Jesus is building and the gates of Hades will not prevail against? You mean the church that is the temple of the Spirit of God? And somehow the New Testament has left us in the dark? Are you telling me that you don't believe the Scripture is sufficient?"

Or you may run into somebody in the field of psychology, as I did at a conference where I was preaching on the authority of the Word of God and the Bible as the means for dealing with every spiritual issue. One pastor raised his hand and said, "I believe that the Bible is the only source for truth which sanctifies, but some people can't even get themselves in a position to be sanctified until they are 'jump-started' by a therapist."

What about Scripture? Does philosophy offer us the necessary groundwork to jump-start ethics? Does psychology offer us the necessary foundation to jump-start sanctification? Just what does the Bible offer?

> The law of the Lord is perfect, restoring the soul; The testimony of the Lord is sure, making wise the simple. The precepts of the Lord are right, rejoicing the heart; The commandment of the Lord is pure [literally, clear], enlightening the eyes. The fear of the Lord is clean, enduring forever; The judgements of the Lord are true; they are righteous altogether (Psalm 19:7-9, NASB).

Those are statements about sufficiency. The apostle Paul, in 2 Corinthians 3:5 (KJV), said, "Our sufficiency is of God." Jesus said, in John 17:17 (KJV) [Father,] "Sanctify them through thy truth: thy word is truth." In 1 Corinthians 2:13 (KJV), the Spirit of God opens to us the Word of God "not in words which man's wisdom teacheth, but which the Holy Spirit teacheth." And because of that, verse 15 says, we can judge, and appraise, and evaluate all things because we have the mind of Christ.

With that background from some New Testament texts that are familiar to us, I want us to look at Psalm 19. *There are six statements in those three verses.* Each verse is a couplet. Each of those six statements has three elements. There are *six titles for Scripture*: it is called the *law* of the Lord, the *testimony* of the Lord, the *precepts* of the Lord, the *commandments* of the Lord, the *fear* of the Lord, and the *judgments* of the Lord. With each of those titles, the covenant name of Yahweh is repeated. That is to remind us, without any kind of equivocation, that God is the author. What you have, then, is Scripture looked at in six facets, as a diamond might be viewed. Scripture is all of this. It is *law, testimony, precept, commandment, fear, and judgment.* Those are just different ways to view Scripture.

Second, there are *six characteristics of Scripture.* It is *perfect, sure, right, clear, clean, and true.* Scripture then has *six benefits: it restores the soul, makes wise the simple, rejoices the heart, enlightens the eyes, endures forever,* and the last one, literally, produces *comprehensive righteousness.* Six titles, six characteristics, and six benefits.

Here then, in these verses, you have comprehensive statements made on the absolute sufficiency of the Word of God. Let's take them one at a time.

Statement number one: *The law of the Lord is perfect, restoring or converting the soul.* This views Scripture as law, and certainly it is that. To give it another title, we might say divine instruction is the operating manual of the human being. Scripture is God's giving man an explanation of how he is to live. It is instruction for man's conduct. As such, He says it is perfect.

The first time I studied Psalm 19 I decided I was going to find out what that word meant, so I spent an afternoon, maybe three hours, chasing around my Hebrew lexicons and looking at every source I had to try to discern what the word *perfect* meant to the Hebrews. After three hours or so I found out that what it really means is "perfect," which was a bit discouraging, to be honest with you. I suppose that's why James called it "the perfect law." But it is set here in contrast to the imperfect and flawed reasonings of men. Scripture is perfect, implying that man's wisdom is imperfect. But what does *perfect* mean to the Hebrew? The best lexicon definition I read is this: It means all-sided, so as to cover completely all aspects of something. "Scripture is comprehensive" is what it is saying. It is not so much the idea of being flawless, as opposed to being flawed, but it is the idea of being complete, as opposed to being incomplete. It is comprehensive, and the benefit of that is noted here: restoring the soul. The Hebrew word for *restoring* could be reviving, restoring, refreshing, or as the most familiar translation puts it, converting. The best translation is "totally transforming."

The Scripture, divine instruction for men, is so complete and comprehensive that it can totally transform the soul, *nefesh,* a very familiar word to anybody who studies the Old Testament. It's translated in my English version twenty-two different ways. Now that will tell you that not any one word gets at it; sometimes life, sometimes person, sometimes heart, sometimes soul, sometimes being—twenty-two different English words. What it means is the inner person, the complete inner person. Now let's put it together. *The Scripture is so comprehensive that it can totally transform the whole inner person. What an immense statement!*

I think the primary significance of that statement is to affirm the regenerating power of Scripture, its saving capability. It is much as what Peter said, "Being born again, not of corruptible seed, but of incorruptible, by the word of God" (1 Pet. 1:23, KJV). Paul said, "For I am not ashamed of the gospel of Christ: for it is the power of God unto salvation" (Rom. 1:16, KJV). It is the Word that powerfully transforms. Second Timothy 3:15 says it is the Word, the Scriptures, which are able to make you wise unto salvation. The Word is the power that transforms. I believe that with all my heart. That's why, whenever I step into a pulpit, I preach the Word.

I was at a meeting in Sebring, Florida, and a nice-looking young man came up to me, probably about thirty-five, and said, "Can I talk to you for a few moments? I want to share a testimony with you that I think will encourage you." I said, "Certainly." He said, "My name is Tim Ervolina, and I am a fifth-generation Jehovah's Witness. My father is in charge of the Jehovah's Witnesses for this area. I am also very involved; I am the trainer for all of the JW pastors in Florida. I travel around, and I teach them how to do their ministry. Just a few weeks ago I was driving in my car and I turned the radio on and you were preaching. I was listening to you—I didn't know who you were—and I heard you say 'Jesus is God.' In fact, you read a few Bible verses that supported the thought that Jesus is God, and I reached over and turned the radio off. I said, 'That's a lie.' Then curiosity got me and I turned it back on. You kept preaching that Jesus is God. That was on a Monday. Since I was in the same general area I listened to you every day that week. On Friday you said you were going to continue the series next week, so I have to tell you that I listened every day the next week. For ten days you kept opening the Scripture, showing that Jesus is God. On Friday night I was in a motel, and I got down on my knees and said, 'Jehovah, if you came into the world in the form of Jesus Christ, show me, and I will commit my life to Christ.' Before the dawn of that Saturday morning I was born again. It was the power of the Word of God that I could not debate. For the last four weeks I have been going back to all the Jehovah's Witness churches and giving them all the gospel, and telling them all that Jesus is God."

I thought to myself after talking with him, *How do you reach a JW? How subtle do you have to be? How programmed do you have to be to understand all that he understands?* How about just shouting at him for ten days, "Jesus is God!" Not very subtle. He said to me, "Pray for my father and my mother; pray for my wife and my two sons. They are all JWs." Within five months I got a letter from him. He said, "Thank you for your prayers. My mother and father are converted, my wife is converted, both my sons are in Christ." That's the power of the Word.

Let me tell you one that will come close to home. One Sunday afternoon I had an appointment with a man who is a medical doctor. He had been visiting our church. He called my secretary on Friday and said, "I want to come in and see John MacArthur if I can. I have a real problem." At four o'clock on a Sunday afternoon, before the evening service, he walked into my office. He took my hand and said, "My name is Steve. I need help. I am damned." I said, "You are damned?" He said, "Yeah, I have never been in a church in my life until the last four weeks, and I came to your church. You've been doing a series on 'Delivered to Satan,' and that's me. I'm damned." I said, "Why do you say that?" He said, "I kill babies for a living. I run a clinic in L.A. Last year we did nine million dollars worth of abortions. If a woman comes in and doesn't have a good reason, I give her one. Furthermore, my life is a mess. I left my first wife, married my second wife, left my second wife, and I'm living with a woman who is not my wife. I've been in psychiatric counseling for a year, and I'm having severe financial problems. To add to that, I'm Jewish, and I'm not supposed to believe anything you say. But my life is a wreck. Can you help me?"

In all honesty I said to him, "No. I can't help you. But I know someone who can. Jesus Christ can transform your life if you will expose yourself to His truth." He said, "Well, I will do whatever you ask me, but remember, I am a man of science; I must have proof." I will never forget that statement. I said, "Fine." I reached over to my desk and picked up a Bible. It happened to be a New International Version. I opened it and said, "See this book called 'John'? Read it. Just take it home, keep reading it until you know who Jesus is and why He came. No tapes, no books, just read this." He said, "That's all?" I said, "Just keep reading it until you know who Jesus Christ is." He tucked that Bible under his arm and went away and I prayed for him, because I know this: It is the Spirit of God alone who can quicken the heart. And He can only quicken the heart to respond to the truth when the truth is perceived.

Thursday I get a phone call. "This is Steve. I need to see you again." Sunday, same time, he walks in like I wasn't even there, walks right by me, sits on the couch, and says, "I know who He is. He is God! Jesus is God!" I said, "You're a Jew. Your two kids were bar mitvahed. You don't even believe in Jesus Christ. You're telling me at this age (probably 48 years old or so), in one week you are now convinced Jesus is God?" He said, "He has to be God. Only God could do what He did and say what He said. And do you know what else He did? He rose from the dead! And you know what amazed me? He did it so fast! Only God could do that." I said to him, "Do you know why He came?" He said, "Oh, yeah, I know why He came. He came to die for my sins." I said, "How did you know that?" He flipped through the pages of his Bible and said, "See this book called 'Romans'? I read that, too." He had all this red underlining through Romans. I said, "I'm overwhelmed. Does this have any implications in your life?" He said, "Yeah, I spent this afternoon writing my resignation letter to the clinic. I called my wife, and I invited her to church. She's meeting me at church tonight."

He hasn't yet come to that commitment to Christ, but he's making moves. He's out of that business, he's back with his wife, and I'm his conscience, just poking away at him. I believe he will come to know Christ. It is the power of the Word of God that can totally transform the whole person. I'm just so convinced of that. I'm not concerned about the packaging; I'm concerned about the truth.

Second, the psalmist says, in verse 7, *"the testimony of the* Lord *is sure, making wise the simple." Testimony* describes Scripture as God's own witness, God's own personal testimony. He's revealing Himself. Certainly that's true of Scripture. It's not only a manual on human behavior, instruction for how man is to live, but it's also the revealed truth about God. And He says it is sure, as opposed to that which is human, which is unsure. The Scripture is unmistakable, it is unwavering, it is reliable, it is able to be trusted. It is a more sure word of prophecy (2 Pet.1;19), Peter says, than any human experience. Then I love this: He says the Scripture, which is reliable and trustworthy, makes simple people wise.

The Hebrew language is very concrete. It is not an abstract language like Greek. Usually in Hebrew when you see a word that might appear to be abstract, like the word *simple,* it has a pretty concrete foundation. In fact, the word for simple here is a wonderful word, which means "an open door." A simple-minded person, to a Jew, was somebody who had the door to his brain open. We would call it open-minded. The Hebrew would call it simple-minded. The Jew would say, "Look, if you are open-minded, close the door, will you?" You have a door on your house to keep some things in, like children and heat, and some things out, like robbers and cold. The same thing is true in your mind. You must learn when to close it and keep some things in and some things out. A simple-minded person was a naive person, without the ability to discriminate, lacking wisdom, lacking skill in discernment, uninformed, inexperienced. Scripture takes the naive, the person with the open mind, and helps him close the door. It makes him actually wise— *shakam* in Hebrew, a wonderful word meaning "skilled in all aspects of living." It takes the naive, uninitiated, ignorant, uninformed person and makes that person skilled in all aspects of holy living.

You see, to the Hebrew, wisdom wasn't the *sophos* of the Greeks, meaning *what they knew.* Wisdom *was what you did.* And if you knew something and didn't do it, you were the biggest fool of all. To the Hebrew the word *shakam* meant the ability to make right decisions, and particularly to make right decisions at the crisis moments of life. It was the practical matter of living life with all spiritual skill. The Word of God, then, is adequate for every issue of life.

Third, verse 8 says, *"The precepts of the Lord are right, rejoicing the heart."* This views Scripture as divine precepts, or to say it another way, principles to make life meaningful and joyful and fulfilling and satisfying and happy. He says the precepts of the Lord, Scripture viewed as principles, are right—not right as opposed to wrong, but the actual word means "a right path" as opposed to taking a wrong path. In other words, Scripture gives you the map so you can get through the maze of life, through the confounding, convoluted, difficult issues of life. Scripture is your only true guide, in the hands of the indwelling Holy Spirit, to lead you through the maze of confusion. And it leads you where? To joy: It "rejoices the heart."

That's such a great concept. Jeremiah 15:16 (KJV) says, "Thy words were found, and I did eat them; and thy word was unto me the joy and rejoicing of mine heart." John, in writing his first epistle, said, "These things write we unto you, that your joy may be full" (1 John 1:4, KJV). Scripture is given to us to show us the path of life. In walking through the maze of the mine-field of life we find true joy—not from self-indulgent activities, not from self-gratification, not from mystical science of the mind, but through the Word of God. In fact, Jesus put it this way: "Happy are those who hear the word or God and obey it" (Luke 11:28, TEV). "Happy is the man who listens to me," it says in Proverbs 8:34 (RSV). Do you remember the fellowship of the burning heart in Luke 24:32 (NIV), the road to Emmaus? "Were not our hearts burning within us while he talked with us on the road and opened the Scriptures to us?" This is the burning, exhilarating, thrilling joy, such as that which came to the eunuch who, after his conversion, went on his way rejoicing. Scripture is the source of transformation. Scripture is the source of wisdom and skill in all matters of holy living. And Scripture is the place where you find the path through the maze of confusing things, the mine-field of the world, and the path is the path of joy.

Fourth statement, in verse 8: *"The commandment of the Lord is pure [clear], enlightening the eyes."* Boy, do we want enlightenment! Boy, do we need it! What does he say? The commandment of the Lord—His divine decrees—are not suggestions. This is an authoritative, sovereign, binding, non-optional set of demands by God on man. Scripture is mandatory. And Scripture, he says, is clear. "Wayfaring men, though fools, shall not err" (Isa. 35:8, KJV). Even a child, even babes can understand it, Jesus said. The word *clear* here is better than pure; it means lucid, easy to see, easy to understand. It gives clear direction, it enlightens the murky darkness, in contrast to the muddled musings of men who try to solve unsolvable problems with no standard, no plumb line. The Word gives us understanding in the dark things.

Through my years of ministry as a pastor, I have dealt with people in the dark and bleak times of life. I am reminded of families I know who have children with cystic fibrosis. In my own family, I have three sisters with double mastectomies. I have lived through all of that, I understand all of that, but I understand it with an enlightened understanding because I understand that I have three sisters in Christ who are headed for Glory. But I deal with people, as you do too, who don't have that understanding, and they have nothing but the blackness of the reality. They don't understand the future, therefore they can't understand the present. They have no hope. They don't experience the comfort of the Scriptures. They don't know what Psalm 119 means when it says, "I hope in thy word" (Psa. 119:114, KJV). Scripture opens up all the dark things and makes them light.

John Romanosky and his wife, Nora, wonderful missionaries, served the Lord for many years in Brigham City, Utah, at the Brigham City Bible Church, trying to win Mormons to Christ. They had a little church, a very difficult ministry. John and Nora had two beautiful daughters and a wonderful son. They decided to come to Southern California a couple of years ago. John said, "I want to bring my family down to a big church. I want to enroll my oldest daughter in The Master's College. And we are going to have a family vacation in Southern California. We are going to bring two foreign exchange students from Italy. We are bringing them because they are not saved, and we want to win them to Christ on our family vacation."

So John and Nora and the two beautiful girls, one a senior and the other a sophomore in high school, and their son in the ninth grade, and the two foreign exchange students piled in the big family station wagon and came to Southern California. They went on a

Saturday out to the college and enrolled their oldest daughter in school. They left the college, and they were driving along, and stopped at a red light. Inadvertently, somehow John pulled out against the red light. A truck coming down a hill, full speed, hit the car broadside right behind John and Nora. The impact catapulted his daughters, who were in the back, out the window, against the curb, and both of them were killed instantly. The three boys wound up with severe internal injuries in a hospital. The car went up in flames. John and Nora had their glasses shattered, their Bibles incinerated; their shoes went through the windshield. They were smashed and banged around in the front but received no severe injuries. What started out as a happy, wonderful family vacation ended in an unthinkable holocaust. Two dead daughters in the street, and these young men splattered all over everywhere, the car in flames. My son Mark happened to be coming by, called for the ambulance, and came and told me.

As fast as I could I got to John and I said, "John, I don't know what to say. I don't have the words, but I just want to ask you, what are you thinking?" I will never forget what he said to me. Now remember, this is after years and years of ministry in the hard, hard place, where you might kind of think maybe God would give you some special consideration. John said, "My first thought is, 'It's a dream, and I'll wake up and it won't be true.' But I know that's not the case." Then through his tears he said, "My second thought is this: 'Isn't God good, isn't He gracious, that He took my two daughters, who love Him, and spared those two unsaved boys." That's seeing in the light, isn't it? That darkness was made light for him. It was about a week later he stood in front of our congregation and gave testimony to the grace of Christ. They stayed for weeks until their son healed. The parents came from Italy, and the boys healed. During all that time he was sharing Christ with those two boys, and they made professions of faith in Him. Eventually he took his wife and his one son and went back to Brigham City. In a few months he wrote me a letter and said, "We have a more fruitful ministry now than we have ever had, because no one can quite understand our trust in the Lord." I can live life if I can see like that.

One day the neurosurgeon called me in and said, "Mr. MacArthur, your son has a brain tumor. It could be fatal." I don't want to hear this. My son loves Christ with all his heart. He's a big, strapping, athletic guy, a verbal communicator, a leader. I'm saying, "Lord, you got the right kid? You sure this is the one?" But I began to fast and pray. The Lord took me through nine days of fasting and praying for Mark while I drove him to the Frank Norris Cancer Clinic for non-invasive tests to try to determine what this thing was. At first I am praying that God will spare him, and by about day six I am praying that God will take him—the Lord just turned my heart. Why leave him here if he can be there, right? Through that whole catharsis the light of eternal glory and reality allowed me to release my son to the Lord. And it enhanced my prayer life in a profound way. In fact, it ended in a most unique way. It was a Wednesday and a lady knocked on my door. I had devoted myself to pray, but felt hungry for the first time in eight or nine days. I think the Lord impressed upon my heart that it was time for the fast to end. But I did not want to go to a fast-food place, not to end something significant like this. This lady knocked on my door—she had never been in my office before and she's never been there since—and said, "I was just thinking about you, pastor. I knew you were in the church waiting for the Wednesday evening service, and I made you a sandwich." I don't know if I said anything, I was so shocked. When she put the little bologna sandwich on my desk and walked away, I thought, "God's involved in my life when He delivers the sandwich to end the fast." The next morning the doctor called and said, "I have good news for you! We are all convinced the tumor is epidermoid. It's inconsequential—it's not even going to grow. Don't worry about it." And we haven't. It has stayed the same, and he's doing great!

As I look at that, I can't understand how a parent would face that with no hope. "Why did you give me this child, just to do this to me? To give me such a profound love for him and them just rip him out of my life?" The Word of God is light in dark places. It enlightens the eyes.

Fifth, in verse 9: *"The fear of the Lord is clean, enduring forever."* Fear pictures the Bible as a manual on worship. It's our instruction on understanding that God is awesome. It is a book about how to worship, and we are true *worshipers*. As such, it is clean, without error, without corruption, without evil, and without stain. Simply stated, it then has to be from God, because everything man touches gets blighted. *Tahor* is the root in the Hebrew. It has the idea of the absence of impurity, defilement, filthiness, or imperfection. It is unsullied. Psalm 12:6 says that the words of the Lord are pure words, like silver tested in a furnace seven times. As such, it lasts forever. What makes things die? Sin. Corruption. This doesn't die. It is permanently relevant. It doesn't need redaction; it doesn't need updating; it doesn't need contemporizing or acculturation. It never needs any help. It is a permanent and enduring and lasting source of instruction, because it is hallowed and holy and separate and pure.

And then lastly, he says about Scripture, *"It is the judgment of the Lord which is true; it produces comprehensive righteousness."* This depicts Scripture as divine adjudications from the Judge of all the earth, verdicts from the bench, it is God's verdict on human life and destiny, divine determinations by the Judge of all the earth from the heavenly bench. He says Scripture, as such, is true. What a great and profound statement! So simple. It's true! I wish we could just tell that to our culture. You want truth? It's here!

Paul put it this way: They are "ever learning and never able to come to the knowledge of the truth" (2 Tim. 3:7, KJV). And here we Christians are, not many noble, not many mighty, we are not the elite of the world, we are just common folks. Yet we can walk into any kind of a situation, no matter how academic it is, and say, "Ladies and gentlemen, I am here to tell you the truth."

I am invited to speak on university campuses. California State University department of philosophy invited me in. I love it! They wanted me to come in and speak on Christian sex ethics. Well, there couldn't be anything more unpopular to a bunch of college kids than Christian sex ethics. I went in there and this guy was a former rabbi, teaching philosophy, and he just loved to chew up fundamentalists. So I knew I had to be kind of prepared. I said, "First of all, ladies and gentlemen, I want to thank Dr. Kramer for letting me come in. I just want to tell you, I am here to tell you the truth—the truth about everything—the truth about life, death, love, the truth about right and wrong, the truth about how the world started, how it's going to end." I just started this little scenario, and you could just see them mumbling to each other, "It's incredible. This guy is off his rocker!" I said, "I can tell you why you are here and what you are for and where you are going and how you got here. I can tell you how to have a meaningful marriage, a meaningful family, how to have a meaningful friendship, how to make the tough, moral, ethical decisions." You see, they don't ever find the truth, because if they find the truth, class is over.

Finally, when I finished saying all this, I said, "Now, even though I've said all that, none of you are going to accept what I say. I can tell you the truth about morality and all that, but you are not going to accept it. There's no way you are going to accept what I say."

One big guy said, kind of defiantly, "How do you know that? How do you know we won't?" And I knew I had reversed the roles.

"Because you can't accept this truth: There's a prerequisite." He said, "What is it?" I said, "You must have a personal knowledge of the true God through His Son Jesus Christ or you will never accept this." Somebody else asked, "Well, how do you have that?" I said, "Good, now let's get to the real issue." And we spent the rest of the time on the gospel! In college I took advanced philosophy, European philosophy, and all that, and I'd fuddled around. I still read Paul Johnson and try to stay up on some of that stuff. But I'm telling you, it was just terrific to walk into that massive amount of chaos and just start nailing the truth, and saying it's in Christ, and summing it all up with, Jesus said, "I am the way, the truth, and the life."

We may not be the elite of the world, but we know the truth. That's a privilege and that is also a responsibility. And what does this truth produce? Comprehensive righteousness, according to verse 9. That's what that last phrase means. It produces comprehensive righteousness for an individual, for a family, for a church, for a nation.

Now, you tell me what people are looking for. Do you think people would like to have their lives changed, or do you think they are blissfully happy the way everything is? Inside, I don't think so. They are riddled with guilt and shame, confusion, hate, disappointment. I think they would like transformation. Not only that, I think they would like to be skilled in all the issues of life. I also think they would like loads of joy. They would like to be able to see clearly the dark things of life that they cannot understand. They would like to find some sort of enduring reality that is not relative to the changing times. And they would like, I believe, the truth. And they would like something that would consummately make them the people they can potentially be. Every cry of the human heart is satisfied in the sufficiency of Scripture.

As a result of that, the psalmist says, in Psalm 19:10 (NASB): [Scripture is] "more desirable than gold, yes than much fine gold; Sweeter also than honey and the drippings of the honeycomb." He says it's our most precious possession and our sweetest pleasure. Then he says, in verse 11, "Moreover, by them Thy servant is warned." It is our greatest possession, it is our greatest pleasure, it is our greatest protector. It warns us. Then he says that in the keeping of the Scripture there is great reward. It is our greatest provider. In verse 12 he says, "Who can discern his errors? Acquit me from hidden faults. Also keep back Thy servant from presumptuous sins." Don't let them rule over me. "Then I shall be blameless, And I shall be acquitted of great transgression." It is our greatest purifier. In light of all that, he sums it up in verse 14 and says, "Let the words of my mouth and the meditation of my heart Be acceptable in Thy sight, O Lord, my rock and my Redeemer." You say, "What does that have to do with Scripture?" Everything. The psalmist knew Joshua 1:8 (NASB): "This book of the law shall not depart from your mouth, but you shall meditate on it day and night, so that you may be careful to do according to all that is written in it; for then you will make your way prosperous, and then you will have success." The psalmist knew that where God wants His children to meditate is on the Scripture. So in verse 14 he was saying, "Let me commit my life to the study and meditation of Scripture."

I have a friend who has a Bible collection. Among the incredible pieces in that collection is a Bible which, the first time I saw it, made me weep. I just stood there like a baby. He has it in a little pulpit, with a cover, which I opened up. It was a very large Bible, coming out of the sixteenth century. I flipped it open, and immediately I realized that the bottom half of it had been wet. You know how a book gets when it gets soaked and all the pages get kind of wrinkled. As I looked closer I could see that the bottom half of the page had a pink tint to it. I said, "What happened to this?" He told me the story of Christians in England at that time who were killed for their faith in Christ. In this case, and in others, before they would execute the Christian they would slit him somewhere and fill a bowl with his blood, then take the Bible and throw it in there. This Bible had the name of the man in the front and a lot of little things written in there like you and I write in our Bibles, very personal, and bathed in his own blood. I just stood there and kept turning the pages as the tears ran out of my eyes, because suddenly I realized the price that some have paid to put this in my hand. People have given their lives for this Book.

God is not asking us to do that. He's not saying, "Would you please be a dead sacrifice?" He's saying, "Would you please be a living one?" I think if there's anything that we must do, it's the *only* thing we can do, and that is to bring to this generation this Book. Every preacher, every teacher, every Christian needs to start proclaiming God's Word loud and clear.

Endnotes

[1]Thomas Watson, *A Body of Divinity* (Edinburgh: Banner of Truth, 1965), 27.

[2]John F. MacArthur, Jr., *Our Sufficiency in Christ* (Dallas: Word, 1991).

Medicine and Morality Without God

By Franklin E. Payne

We are experiencing the largest epidemic in the history of both the United States and of the world. Predictions are that 330,000 people in the United States will have died of AIDS by the end of 1995. Some 80,000 children will be orphaned by the year 2000 because one or both of their parents will have died of AIDS.[1]

However, these numbers, staggering as they are and quite personal to all of us, pale beside the numbers worldwide. The World Health Organization estimates that from 40 to 100 million people around the world will be infected with HIV by the turn of the century.

There is something else unique about this epidemic, however, besides its massive numbers. It is a disease of immorality, and it is a disease that has been wrongly managed by medical professionals, and by state "officials." From these characteristics, I get my theme for this chapter. That is, the HIV/AIDS epidemic is a paradigm for the direct correlation between morality and health among individuals, society, and the state.

In this anti-intellectual age that unfortunately includes Christians as well as unbelievers, the worst approach is to begin with definitions. However, you will not understand much of what follows without those definitions. And I want you to understand.

The first definition concerns the word "state." When I use "state," I am including all levels of government, not just a state like Tennessee or Georgia. I am referring to the people who make laws and who enforce them.

The second definition is more a description of two names, "experts" and "officials." Whenever I write about HIV/AIDS, I put "experts" and "officials" within quote marks. I do that because they may have the status of an official or expert, but many of their judgments are those of fools rather than experts. Lest you think me harsh, I remind you that the biblical concept of "fool" is a person who fails to acknowledge God and His truth. "The fool" has said in his heart, 'There is no God'" (Ps. 14:1). Fools, rather than officials, have legislated and enforced the rules and laws for the AIDS epidemic, and their advice has been foolish, as we will see.

HIV/AIDS: A Spectrum of Diseases

The third definition is also a description. To use "HIV/AIDS" repeatedly will be tiresome for both you and me, thus I will use one or the other according to the context. However, the relationship of HIV and AIDS is important to an understanding of this epidemic.

"HIV" stands for human immunodeficiency virus, which is commonly referred to as the "AIDS virus." It is the first retrovirus of its type to infect humans. Since a second such retrovirus has been discovered, the scientific literature refers to the AIDS virus as HIV-1. I will leave off the "one" to avoid redundancy. (HIV-2 has not infected large numbers of people and probably will not.)

HIV infection is best understood as a spectrum. When a person first becomes infected, he may or may not experience a "flu-like" illness within a few weeks. Usually, this episode has nothing about it to alarm the person that something much more significant is happening within his body. Symptoms differ from one person to another but may include a sore throat, muscle aches, fever, rash, and headache.

Lymph node swelling may or may not be prominent. If it is, this finding may be the only indication that something other than the flu is present. The illness may last a few days or two to three weeks, but it resolves without treatment. (Large glands in a teenager may be infectious mononucleosis, a disease more significant than most cases of the flu but far less significant than HIV.)

Then the virus enters a quiet period for several years. Just how long it may remain quiet is variable, but we know that it may be dormant for ten years or more. During this time, the infected person experiences his usual health. Inside his body, however, the HIV is slowly destroying his T-cells (white blood cells that assist other white blood cells, the B-lymphocytes, to make antibodies). At some point during this latent period, the person may develop lymph nodes that are quite large, but not necessarily painful or tender. At this stage, the HIV is beginning to compromise the body's defenses.

The T-cells are gradually reduced in number until the person's resistance is overcome, and signs and symptoms appear. These symptoms may be due to "opportunistic" infections; that is, infections that rarely infect people with normal immune systems. Or, symptoms may be due to the HIV itself. These signs and symptoms include thrush (a fungal infection of the mouth), inflammation of the gums, herpes Type I lesions (blisters that are extremely painful), diarrhea, fever and sweats, and severe weight loss (the "wasting syndrome"). Neurologic symptoms such as numbness, muscle dysfunction, and confusion may occur. This stage may be called AIDS-Related Complex (ARC). It is not yet AIDS, even though the person may be severely ill and die before progressing to AIDS.

AIDS is the final and severe stage of HIV infection and also consists of opportunistic infections. One common infection is *Pneumocystis carinii* pneumonia, a parasitic infection of the lungs. Other severe infections include toxoplasmosis, various intestinal parasites, generalized fungal infections, and unusual strains of tuberculosis. A rare form of cancer, *Kaposi's sarcoma,* typically affects the skin, but growths may occur on almost any organ in the body. Lymphoma, a type of leukemia, may occur as well. Without treatment (with zidovudine [AZT] or other anti-viral drug), one-half of all patients will die within the first year after the diagnosis of AIDS is made.

The importance of understanding this spectrum of HIV/AIDS is that AIDS is the only stage of this disease that is required to be reported in every state. (A few states require the reporting of any stage of HIV infection.) Thus, the only accurate numbers to track this epidemic are those at the end of this spectrum. The numbers of those who are infected with HIV but who have not progressed to AIDS are estimated from a large variety of studies from clinics and sub-sets of the general population. This estimate is now one million. Virtually 100 percent of these will eventually get AIDS, unless they die of another illness or injury before they progress to the stage of AIDS.

Even the reporting of AIDS cases is not straightforward. AIDS was first defined by the Centers for Disease Control (CDC) in 1982. The definition was revised in August 1987. This change was broader than the original definition and comprises 27 percent of the current total of AIDS cases. In other words, without this definition change, more than 70,000 fewer AIDS cases would have been reported to date.

Then, beginning in January 1993, the definition was expanded again. With this further broadened definition, the CDC expects an 80 percent increase in the reported AIDS cases in 1993 over 1992 or close to 100,000 cases. The numbers will decrease in subsequent years because they will only include newly reported cases of AIDS, whereas the 1993 cases will include a pool of HIV-infected people who could not have been classified as AIDS cases until the definition change.

So, in a sense, reported AIDS cases include apples (the first definition), oranges (the second definition), and now, I guess, lemons (the third definition) for the sour taste one gets when dealing with such a jumble of statistics!

Without the change in definition in 1987, reported AIDS cases would have fallen quite short of projections made prior to the change. Although I don't believe the CDC made the change to "shore up" their projections, the effect was indeed that their projections were made accurate by this definition change.

My own opinion agrees with that of Dr. Robert Redfield,[2] who heads the U.S. Army's task force on HIV/AIDS. Several years ago the CDC should have made any stage of HIV infection a reportable disease. With such statistics, everyone would be much more certain about just what numbers of HIV infections are present in the United States, and more importantly, how many new infections are occurring each year.

Thus, reported AIDS cases still are the tip of the iceberg that we can see. HIV infection that has not progressed to AIDS is a much larger body that is more or less out of sight of most statistics.

Let's Shift Gears for a Moment

Once again, the HIV/AIDS epidemic is a paradigm for the direct correlation between morality and health among individuals, society, and the state.

Most experts will tell you that the AIDS epidemic began in the late 1970s and continued into the early 1980s. The first AIDS cases appeared in 1981, but allowing for the slow progression of the HIV, these people were actually infected several years earlier. The tens of thousands of AIDS cases reported since then also became infected many years earlier. In that sense, the AIDS epidemic is less than two decades old. From the first reported cases, only twelve years.

However, the AIDS epidemic actually began with what Francis Schaeffer called "post-Christian America." One can trace a decline in the reliance of the American people on biblical truth from the birth of this country, the late 18th century. In the early colonies, a staunch, biblical Christianity existed.

Not only did many immigrants come to the New World for religious freedom, the early colonies experienced the Great Awakening. There were the Puritans of Massachusetts, the Congregationalists of New England, the Methodists evangelized by John Wesley, and of course, the Baptists were growing in numbers! There is no doubt in my mind of the biblical influence in early America.

Pre-constitutional America experienced the height of biblical influence in our history. The Declaration of Independence, however, shows the beginning of a transition. In English and Scottish law, a phrase for freedom was "life, liberty, and (the ownership of) property." The Declaration, however, while acknowledging the Creator, changed the phrase to "life, liberty, and happiness." Without the possession of property, the Sixth Commandment cannot be violated; a subtle but nevertheless powerful departure from biblical government had begun.

The U. S. Constitution shows another profound change. The power of government as an agent of "certain inalienable rights" endowed by the "Creator" in the Declaration became the agent of "We the people" in the Preamble of the Constitution. Thus, by its literal reference, the authority for federal government is humanism, not biblical Christianity.

Please give me some "literary license" in this very brief historical review. I am not a studied historian, but I am convinced that what I have stated is based in historical fact. Many authors have written on these subjects. However, might we at least agree that in our past both the government and its people have increasingly departed from a biblical Christianity?

Other marked changes in Americans' religious beliefs occurred in the 19th century, but I skip over those. In the early 20th century, Bible-believers found it necessary to defend orthodox, traditional, and biblical Christianity against the increasing liberal views. The "fundamentals" were written and hence the term "fundamentalist" was born.

Two aspects of the same phenomenon should be recognized in this event. First, there existed an increasing number and influence of atheists and agnostics. Second, the identification of liberal and conservative was becoming clearer. The conservatives held to biblical beliefs. Liberals not only departed from biblical beliefs, but began to attack them.

The next event that we jump to is the sexual revolution of the 1960s. "Free love" and "open marriages" were "in." We heard, "If it feels good, do it." Another giant leap was taken from traditional and biblical beliefs in sexual license and liberty.

That's the spiritual and moral history that preceded the AIDS epidemic in something smaller than a nutshell! However, there were parallels in medicine and science as well.

Medical Practice and Immorality

I begin our pertinent medical history with the early 20th century. Prior to that time, it had little organization, formal education, or state licensure. Little formal research was done. However, with the rise of physics, chemistry, and other sciences, medical "science" was born. Formal education and licensure requirements were devised and implemented. An "orthodoxy" of medicine, if you will, followed.

Causes of disease, especially infectious diseases, were understood for the first time and effective measures brought to bear against them. Within this development, public health measures came into existence. Typhoid fever, spread through contaminated drinking water, was virtually eliminated. Quarantines were instituted when thought necessary to prevent exposure of noninfected people.

In the 1930s, perhaps as a prelude to the sexual revolution of the 1960s, syphilis was spreading rampantly. At that time, no effective treatment was available. With great effort, however, Dr. Thomas Parran, the surgeon general, began to mobilize public attitudes and public health measures against syphilis.[3] Public attitudes were molded by a clear understanding of how syphilis was transmitted and what people should do to avoid being infected with it.

Public health measures included routine testing and contact tracing. Testing was broad, but not universal. Physicians tested whenever they suspected syphilis in their patients and routinely upon admission to hospitals. Recruits entering the military were tested. Sexually transmitted disease clinics, where anyone could be tested, were started. Testing was required for marriage licenses.

Contact tracing was begun. That is, when a positive test for syphilis was found, the infected person was questioned about his sexual partners and they were contacted to be tested and that person's sexual contacts traced. After penicillin became available to cure syphilis, sexual contacts were treated whether infection could be detected or not, since the incidence of infection was so high and penicillin so effective.

With these efforts, a ten-fold reduction of syphilis cases occurred from 1947 to 1955.[4] With a resurgence of cases in the early 1960s, these same measures were intensified, and cases were reduced but not as strikingly as before. At the time, what was happening may not have been recognizable. However, by hindsight it appears that the sexual revolution was already beginning to overwhelm the public health and medical system.

Medical-Moral Decisions

In 1973, the Supreme Court made abortion legal in its *Roe v. Wade* decision. A lesser-known decision was made by the American Psychiatric Association (APA) that may eventually be as devastating as the abortion decision.

Homosexual activists applied considerable pressure, including physical disruption and takeover of meetings, at successive annual meetings of the APA.[5] Finally, in December 1973, the trustees of the APA voted to remove homosexuality from the Diagnostic and Statistical Manual of Mental Disorders - II (DSM - II) category of diseases.

I call this action a medical-moral decision because psychiatry became legitimate only because of the departure of the American people from biblical Christianity. I don't have space here to defend that position, but suffice it here that homosexuality is a moral/spiritual problem, not a disease, and therefore was never a medical problem in the first place. Because homosexuality is clearly condemned by the Bible,[6] it is not a medical problem. It is a sin problem that needs confession and repentance, not medical help.

We will return to this link between sin and disease, but returning to the APA decision, it was essentially a religious "blessing" on homosexuality that fueled the growth of homosexuality to levels almost unimaginable. Tens and even hundreds of sexual "partners" in a year were, and still are, common. Sections of cities around the world became playgrounds for national and international gay travelers.

With this frenzy of homosexual activity, the stage was set for the AIDS epidemic. The AIDS epidemic did not just happen. The fuel was poured out by our cultural and medical heritage. When ignited, we could virtually only watch it burn. Then, when we could have limited its spread, we poured more fuel on the flame instead.

In all candor, HIV might have occurred when it did whether homosexuality had been rampant or not. Where the virus came from is really not known. It seems to have come out of Africa. I personally believe that it is neither a virus new to mankind nor a mutation from an animal virus. It has been here since creation, causing a few cases here and there, and possibly occasional small outbreaks.

Further, such an epidemic could not have been predicted. The same sexual revolution produced a fire storm of other sexually transmitted diseases sufficient to overwhelm the medical profession and devastate both homosexuals and heterosexuals. Who would have thought a new sexually transmitted disease would appear that was far more deadly than anything known before?

What is certain, however, is that the wildfire spread of HIV occurred because of homosexual behaviors. From them, it spread to IV-drug abusers. From them both, it spread to the blood supply, heterosexual partners, and babies in their mothers' wombs. And, thus, we have the AIDS epidemic—the natural (or supernatural) outgrowth of moral and medical failures.

When the AIDS epidemic did appear, the lessons of syphilis control were not implemented. There were new players on the scene: homosexual activists. They screamed, "Discrimination," and "officials'" knees buckled. Strange measures were instituted. Testing became "anonymous" for the first time. Physicians could not routinely test for HIV. In fact, they could not test without the patient's permission and only then after considerable pre- and post-test counseling.

AIDS patients could not be identified on medical wards for the protection of all health care workers. If a health care worker had a needle-stick, the patient on whom the needle was used could not be tested for HIV without the patient's permission.

Something called "universal precautions" that had been only used in special situations with highly infectious patients or to protect patients from infection became the official proclamation of the CDC for the protection of health care workers. That is, all health care workers were supposed to wear gloves, masks, goggles, gowns, and shoe coverings with every patient. All this effort and expense was not to protect the health-care worker, but to protect the identity of the AIDS patient (i.e., homosexual AIDS patient).

Federal and state funding changed also. Within just a few years, money for research and education for AIDS exceeded heart disease and cancer, the two diseases with the most funding for two decades.

HIV/AIDS as a Paradigm

Remember, my theme is that *the HIV/AIDS epidemic is a paradigm for the direct correlation between morality and health among individuals, society, and the state. A corollary would be that the further society and individuals depart from biblical Christianity, the more disease and death they will experience.*

Let me underscore that I am not speaking of all disease. A great deal of disease does not correlate with one's personal or social morality. Thus, I am not saying that all disease is due to immorality, although ultimately it can be traced to the fall of Adam and Eve. However, virtually any correlation between immorality and disease has been removed from American society.

Sexually transmitted diseases by the millions occur each year, but we hear only a small minority calling for abstinence. Physicians and public health clinics treat these diseases without any moral stigma for the people involved. In fact, they do the opposite. With the removal of the fear of pregnancy through birth control and abortion, sexual license is actually encouraged, thereby increasing the spread of sexually transmitted diseases.

Obesity, worry, stress, alcoholism, and drug and tobacco abuse cause disease and early death by the millions in our society. We hear medical solutions, but not moral solutions.

In summary, the situation is this: Until we once again link morality and health, the diseases that we currently experience will only get worse, not better. Or, until we emphasize the responsibility to act morally instead of the right to medical care without limit for everyone, these disease will only increase.

Do you understand what I am saying? Modern medicine, for all its billions in funding, technology, and experience is virtually powerless in the face of these diseases. Medical costs are out of control because morality is out of control. The American people have placed their hope in medicine instead of Jesus Christ. The god of medicine will as surely fail them as any other god.

The AIDS epidemic is no accident. While the specifics of the epidemic may not have been predictable, the seeds for it were sown a long time ago. We "have sown the wind, and . . . shall reap the whirlwind" (Hos.8:7). Health without morality is impossible. An effective approach to medicine without morality is impossible.

Now, very briefly I want to stop preaching and go to meddling, as preachers are fond of saying. How does all of this affect you? Let me begin with these questions: "Why are your insurance premiums so high? Why have the medical insurance programs of some denominations gone bankrupt?"

The answer to both questions is that Christians have approached medical care and insurance in virtually the same way as non-Christians. We have adopted the ways of the world. Rather than being "transformed by the renewing of our minds" with a different approach, we have "conformed to the world" (Rom. 12:2). If the world is bankrupt, is it any wonder that we are also?

Christians worship the god of medicine almost as much as non-Christians. Thus, they pay their "tithes and offerings beyond the tithe" to the god of medicine. Someone has said that one's checkbook reveals that person's heart. Does our checkbook reveal our faith in modern medicine? I believe it does.

Some Commonly Asked Questions

Can HIV be transmitted by "casual contact"? A qualified, "No." In spite of all that you have heard about the survivability of HIV, transmission of HIV by casual contact is very rare if it occurs at all. I do not say that such transmission is impossible, but standard hygiene measures that people ought to take at all times will virtually eliminate the chance of casual infection with HIV.

Is the blood supply safe? Since the screening of blood for HIV began in 1985, there have been only two reported cases of transmission of HIV compared to 2,956 cases prior to such screens. Transfused blood is safer than it has ever been. My advice, however, is to avoid transfusions whenever possible. Not because of HIV, but because of other risks associated with transfusion. One of the benefits to everyone from the AIDS epidemic is that physicians have learned that transfusions can be avoided in many instances where they had been used routinely before. However, I would not hesitate to have a blood transfusion if it were a life or death situation. There is still no substitute for blood!

Is "everyone" at risk for AIDS? Except for health-care workers, HIV is a virus that you have to go looking for. It will not look for you. Chastity for the unmarried, fidelity for the married, and avoidance of IV-drug abuse offers absolute protection against HIV infection outside medical clinics and hospitals.

On this basis, my answer to the question, "Should everyone be tested for HIV?" is that universal screening is not necessary.

And, my answer to the question, "Should HIV/AIDS patients be quarantined?" is no.

Is it safe to go to the dentist? Yes, the five cases of HIV-transmission by the Florida dentist appear to have been something extraordinary. Thousands of other patients treated by HIV-infected dentists have always tested negative for HIV.

Will there ever be a vaccine against HIV? Not before the year 2000, and probably not then. I don't want to doubt modern technology, but I am doubtful that we will ever have one that is widely effective.

A Conclusion

I will point out that we are living out the description of the first chapter of Romans (vv. 18-32, NKJV). We have rampant homosexuality because God "gave them up to uncleanness, in the lusts of their hearts, to dishonor their bodies among themselves.... even their women exchanged the natural use for what is against nature" (Rom. 1:24, 26). And not only are the most vile and wicked behaviors prevalent, but our social and political (and sometimes church) leaders "not only do the same but also approve of those who practice them" (Rom. 1:32).

And, they implement laws to free them to do these things openly and punish those who oppose them. This policy is a complete reversal of early American thought and behavior. Current medical practice fails largely because of this prevalent immorality. Until our society and its medical practitioners recognize that health and morality are linked, the debacle and devastation of disease will continue.

Endnotes

[1]Franklin E. Payne, Jr., *What Every Christian Should Know About the AIDS Epidemic.* Available from Covenant Books, P. O. Box 14488, Augusta, GA 30919, for $11.00 postpaid.

[2]Robert Redfield, "Perspectives on the AIDS Epidemic," presented at the National Conference on HIV–1987, Washington, D.C. Available in transcript from A.S.A.P., P. O. Box 17433, Washington, D.C. 20041.

[3]Ibid.

[4]Duncan W. Clark and Brian MacMahon, *Preventive and Community Medicine* (Boston: Little, Brown, and Company, 1981): 411-415.

[5]Jonas Robitscher, *The Powers of Psychiatry* (Boston: Houghton Mifflin Company, 1980): 170-177.

[6]Leviticus 18:22; 20:13; Romans 1:26-32; 1 Corinthians 6:9-11; 1 Timothy 1:10.

Teens and Sexually Transmitted Diseases

By Joe S. McIlhaney, Jr.

Sex and sexual activity are good things. I want young people to have all the advantages sex can offer. Healthy and good sex results in pleasure, children, and companionship. It is a spark between men and women that helps them enjoy each other. This type of healthy sex occurs only in marriage. My goal is to help young people understand that by delaying sexual activity and sexual intercourse until they are married they are saving for future good goals. I encourage my patients to exercise now so that they will not only feel better now but will also be healthier and feel better in the future. This is the same principle that I would like to get across to teenagers. If they will not have sex now, if they will delay it until they get married, they will greatly improve their chances of having a healthy and fruitful sexual relationship in the future.

Negative Impact of Teen Sex

Should unmarried adolescents have sex? When this question is asked of most adults, they answer, "No." They are uncomfortable with the idea of adolescents having intercourse because they know it can cause trouble for them now and in the future. Unmarried adolescent sexual activity can:

Hurt a person's relationship with his or her mother, father, sisters, and brothers. Many people in our American society are lonely, and part of the loneliness is the separation we feel from our family when secrets are being kept from them. Those secrets can involve a pregnancy that a teenager has produced in his girl friend. It can include an abortion a girl has without telling her parents. We all need a healthy relationship with our family members, both as young people and as we grow older. Unmarried sexual activity can cause a wedge to be driven between a youngster and his or her family.

Hurt self-esteem and emotional health. Premarital sex is especially destructive to the self-esteem of girls. Premarital sex in teenagers, especially with more than one person, has been linked to emotional illnesses in young people.

Damage spiritual health. When a young person acts contrary to his or her faith it can produce tremendous conflict. Most faiths say that unmarried people should avoid sex until they get married. If a person goes contrary to faith, it can produce either a diminishing of faith or conflict with it that can be very unhealthy.

Damage future opportunities. If girls become pregnant, whether or not they have a child or an abortion, their future opportunities are affected.[1] Teenage pregnancy is the top reason for hospitalization of teenage girls, according to the National Center for Health Statistics, 1983. Over one million pregnancies in girls ten to nineteen occur per year.[2] Four hundred thousand of these pregnancies ended in abortion.[3] The National Center for Health Statistics reported in 1990 that 322,000 births occur to unmarried teenagers per year.

Hurt their physical health and fertility, primarily because of sexually transmitted disease. Although all the other reasons in this section for adolescents to avoid sexual activity are important, I believe that in the public arena, especially in schools and public forums, the problem of adolescent health is reason enough to advise teenagers not to have sex until they get married. I believe my reasoning for this will become quite evident in the information that is to follow.

If young people are taught that they should avoid sex until they get married, some adults become critical. Often these are adults who are single and are having sex with a boyfriend or a girl friend. Often they are teachers who are single and having sex with a boyfriend or a girl friend. They may even be homosexuals who do not agree with this recommendation.

Teens and Sexually Transmitted Diseases

I think it is important for these people to realize that sexual activity among teenagers is a different problem than it is for adults. Teenagers are much more susceptible to sexually transmitted disease. In this chapter from this point on, we are talking about adolescent health, which is a major problem for teenagers who are having sex outside of marriage. Although adults are at risk if they have sex outside of marriage, they can choose to do whatever they want to do. In my opinion they should not criticize efforts to teach young people to avoid sex until they get married because this is the only way young people can be safe from the devastating physical damage which can result from unmarried sex.

Teenagers and STD

Teenagers are far more likely to be infected with sexually transmitted disease and to be damaged by those diseases than adults.

The cervix of a teenage girl has a lining which is more susceptible to STD germs. A large zone of columnar epithelium exists on the girl's cervix, and this type of epithelium is more susceptible to being infected by the bacteria and viruses of sexually transmitted disease.

Teenagers have more menstrual cycles which occur without ovulation. Actually, in the first two years after a girl begins having periods she will often have a period without ovulation. This causes the cervical mucus to be more fluid in consistency and, therefore, more permeable to germs, allowing her to be infected more easily.

Teenagers have lower levels of antibodies against infection in their bodies. Adults have been exposed to many, many types of germs and generally have a high level of antibodies. Teenagers do not have these levels and are, therefore, much more likely to be infected when exposed to germs than are adults.

If teenagers start having sex, they have more sexual partners. Apparently, when a teenager starts a lifestyle of sexual intercourse, he or she adopts a mentality of relating to the opposite sex by having intercourse—even when they leave one partner and move to another one. The Centers for Disease Control showed that if adolescents started having sex before the age of eighteen, at the time they were interviewed 70 percent of them had had two or more sexual partners and 45 percent had had four or more sexual partners. This was compared with people who began having intercourse after the age of nineteen. Only 20 percent of these people had had two or more sexual partners, and only 1 percent had had four or more sexual partners.[4] The importance of this is that the more sexual partners a person has, the more likely he or she is to be infected by sexually transmitted disease. There is a strong correlation between the number of sexual partners and infection with these diseases.

A new phenomenon has occurred during the last 30 years. Until 1960 sex was primarily confined to marriage. Although some people did have sex outside of marriage, most people did not have sex until married and then had sex only in that marriage relationship. Starting about 1960 the sexual revolution changed all that. For the past 30 years we have seen a sexual mixing that had never occurred in the United States. It is common to see studies which show that sexually active teenagers have had five or ten sexual partners. Recently I had a twenty-one-year-old girl tell me that she had twenty-seven sexual partners before she decided that was not the type of lifestyle she wanted.

As a result of this sexual mixing, there has been a progressive emergence of sexually transmitted diseases.

Before 1960	*Syphilis and gonorrhea.* *The only important STDs!*
1976	*Chlamydia first described in association with genital infection. It rarely occurred then; now it is very common.*
1981	*HIV identified. Only a few cases then—now it has killed over 150,000 Americans.*
1984	*Herpes became common. Physician office visits for herpes increased 15-fold from 1966 to 1984.*
1985-1990	*HPV cancers became much more frequent, especially in young people. HPV is now a very common infection. Example: U.C. Berkeley where 6% of sexually active coeds are infected.[5]*

1990	*Antibiotic resistant strains of gonorrhea present in all 50 states.*
1990	*Tubal pregnancies: 400 percent increase in the 1980s.*
1993	*Syphilis at a 40-year high.*
1993	*Pelvic inflammatory disease (PID): One million U.S. women experience this. 16,000-20,000 infections in teenagers.*

This emergence of sexually transmitted diseases has been an astonishing phenomenon. It truly is a legacy of the sexual experimentation of the past thirty years.

Because of the continual emergence of sexually transmitted diseases, there are now twenty-five significant sexually transmitted diseases. More than twelve million people are infected each year in the United States with sexually transmitted disease. It is now estimated that one in five Americans has a sexually transmitted disease and that within the next year one in four Americans will be infected with sexually transmitted disease.

The following are brief summaries of the number of people who are infected with sexually transmitted diseases.

STD Infections

CHLAMYDIA	*3 to 5 million infections per year— 20-40 percent of sexually active singles.*[6]
HUMAN PAPILLOMAVIRUS	*1,500,000 new cases each year in the USA. Up to 46 percent of sexually active singles.*[7]
HERPES	*500,000 new cases each year. 30-40 percent of sexually active singles. 20,000,000 Americans are infected.*[8]

257

AIDS	*1,000,000 new infections in USA in 1990. 1 in 100 at University of Texas, Austin.*[9]
PELVIC INFLAMMATORY DISEASE (PID)	*1,000,000 new cases each year. The most common serious complication of STD.*[10]
GONORRHEA	*1.4 million new infections each year. Resistant forms continue developing.*[11]
SYPHILIS	*130,000 new infections per year. 40-year high. Infects newborns.*[12]
HEPATITIS B	*300,000 cases. Infects newborns.*[13]

This list includes the most significant sexually transmitted diseases. There are other very significant diseases, but because they do not occur so often I did not list them. The other diseases include lymphogranuloma venereum, granuloma inguinale, etc.

Impact of STDs

There are many studies which show the terrible impact of sexually transmitted disease in young people. One of the best examples is pelvic inflammatory disease. PID is a result of chlamydia or gonorrhea infection in a woman's uterus, fallopian tubes, and ovaries. It is said that this is the most common serious effect of a sexually transmitted disease in a person's life. If a girl is sexually active at the age of fifteen, she has a one in eight chance of developing this devastating infection.[14] This risk decreases each year until by the age of twenty-four if a woman is sexually active she has only a one in eighty chance of having PID. If a woman develops PID from chlamydia, she has a 25 percent chance of being sterile. If she has PID because of gonorrhea, she has about a 12 or 13 percent chance of being sterile from only one infection.

If a girl has developed PID as a teenager, she has twice the chance of having a second infection than an older woman has. The problem with this is that if a person has a second episode of PID, she has a 50 percent chance of being sterile if it was caused by chalmydia and a 25 percent chance of being sterile if it was caused by gonorrhea.

If a young girl develops PID it can result in ectopic pregnancies and in infertility. A leading cause of death from pregnancy in all women is ectopic pregnancy, but fifteen- to nineteen-year-olds have the highest mortality risk from ectopics.

Infertility is one of the truly devastating effects of sexually transmitted disease. The percent of married couples who have been affected by infertility has significantly increased for women who are ages twenty to twenty-four. This increase is probably due to sexually transmitted disease. The astounding thing about this is that it is the twenty- to twenty-four-year-old couples who should be the most fertile of all ages. Yet, because of sexually transmitted disease, we are seeing an 11 percent infertility rate in this group.[15]

Twenty years ago it was rare for a teenager or young adult to have cancer of the cervix, vulva, or vagina. It was rare for them to have precancerous changes in these areas. Today, because of the rapid spread of the HPV (human papilloma virus) organism, these precancerous and cancerous changes are very, very common.[16]

What's the Answer?

Every day we read in magazines and newspapers the tremendous strides science is making in the care and treatment of sexually transmitted disease.

I would like to point out that there could be nothing simpler than syphilis to treat. It is easy to find with a simple blood test that is very accurate. It is completely cured by penicillin in its early stages. And, yet, syphilis is at a 40-year high in the United States. Science is not the answer for STDs.

Herpes is an example of the difficulty in developing a vaccine for this type of disease. A vaccine for herpes has been proposed and almost on the market for years—but it is still not available. Herpes can be treated with acyclovir, but this medication costs $1 a pill, and people very often must take two or three of them a day continually, month after month, and year after year for an infection from a sexual relationship.

Chlamydia and gonorrhea can be cured with antibiotics, but the scar and adhesions left are the problems which produce the infertility and ectopic pregnancies already mentioned.

HIV is a very complex organism. I have read that it is a thousand times more complex than herpes. Many researchers feel it will be years before we develop a vaccine or a cure for this infection, even if that is ever possible. It seems unlikely with an infection as complex as HIV that we will solve the problem even if we do have a treatment or vaccine for it. Syphilis is a good example.

It seems very obvious that the answer to this epidemic is not science.

Can we tell young people that if they feel mature and responsible and if they have a partner they care deeply for that they can have sex and be safe? I think we cannot say that.

First, we cannot even tell a teenager that she is safe from pregnancy if she will use birth control pills. M. Klitch pointed out that 6.2 pregnancies per 100 women per year occur with oral contraceptives and that probably more occur in adolescents.[17] Other studies show that with adolescents birth control pill pregnancy rates range up to about 18 percent per year. One reason for this is that teenagers miss, on the average, 2.7 pills per month. But even when they do not miss pills, they are more likely than adults to get pregnant.

Not only can we not tell young people that birth control pills will keep them from pregnancy, we also cannot tell them that condoms will keep them from becoming either pregnant or developing a sexually transmitted disease. The primary association for obstetricians and gynecologists is the American College of Obstetricians and Gynecologists. In a newsletter which was published in March, 1991, the following statement was made:

Condoms and Pregnancy

Despite the high level of technology in Japan, Japanese women still rely heavily on an antiquated system of birth control (condoms). Although the Japanese use condoms more widely than any other people in the world (door-to-door salesmen will provide them), abortion is commonly used as back up for failed contraception. As a result, the country has one of the highest abortion rates of any industrialized, non-communist nation.[18]

If condoms fail this often in preventing pregnancy in a country where they are distributed door-to-door, it seems unrealistic to think that teenagers will be able to use them in such a way that they will not become pregnant or become infected with a sexually transmitted disease. Further, S. Sondheimer made the following statement:

It has to be recognized that there is no completely safe sex. We found, for example, in one year 25% of our patients using condoms conceived: All of them admitted that, on at least one occasion, they did not use a condom.[19]

Dr. Sondheimer is head of the Family Planning Clinic, University of Pennsylvania School of Medicine, Philadelphia, Pennsylvania. This school is one of the outstanding medical schools in the United States. They were counseling with patients one-on-one in a medical facility. If in that environment they could not get people to use condoms any more effectively than they report, how can we expect condoms to protect our teenagers? Especially when we are trying to educate them in a classroom setting with from thirty to fifty students at a time. Further, at Cleveland State University and at three University of California campuses where a combined study was done, it was reported that 5.8% of people said that they always use condoms but 60% said they had never used condoms. The statement was made in this study that, "Despite all the courses on sexual behavior and all the safe-sex advertising on campus, these results were seen."[20]

Many studies show the same thing. In 1990 *The New England Journal of Medicine* reported:

> We conclude that in this population there has been little change in sexual practices in response to new and serious epidemics of STD with the exception of an increase in the use of condoms (which still does not reach 50%).[21]

A startling study done by Dr. Margaret A. Fischl and others stated that 17% of married partners became HIV infected over two years when their partner was HIV infected, even though they knew that the partner was infected and they as a couple used condoms every time.[22]

A study with similar results done by Dr. S. Samuels found that 33% of the women and 37.7% of the men who came through Rutgers University Student Health Center with complaints of a problem in the genital area were culture positive for chlamydia. They found that "Infection rates were equivalent regardless of the contraceptive method. Diaphragm and condom users had infection rates of 44% and 35.7% respectively whereas those using no contraception or oral contraception had infection rates of 44% and 37% respectively."[23]

Will mutually monogamous relationships protect people? No. As a matter of fact, it seems that mutually monogamous relationships in which a person has one sexual partner and then changes to another sexual partner in the next year or two and continues that pattern actually causes people to become infected with sexually transmitted disease. From the same Rutgers study done by Dr. Samuels, they reported that ""The majority of women reported long-term (six months) monogamous relationships. Reported lengthy monogamous relationships were not associated with a low incidence of infection."[24]

We see, therefore, that even when couples were in monogamous relationships they still had just as much infection with chalmydia as if they were not in monogamous relationships and were merely having occasional casual sex.

A similar thing was found by Dr. Minkoff in a study of a group of people who had sexually transmitted disease: "Again, in the study I mentioned that among patients with chlamydia and trichomonas, 80% said they were in a monogamous relationship with people they also trusted were monogamous."[25]

What are the problems with condoms? First, the FDA allows condom manufacturing companies to market condoms if they have three or fewer holes per 1,000. Next, about 7% of the time condoms rupture during use.

More importantly than this, though, is that when a couple has sex with each other for a while, they each become so attached to the other person that they believe this other person could not have an infection which could be dangerous. The couple then stops using condoms and almost universally starts using oral contraceptives to prevent pregnancy. As soon as the condoms are no longer used, the couple has no protection of any kind against sexually transmitted disease. They then are often astounded that they have developed venereal warts, AIDS, or some other sexually transmitted disease as a result of exposure to the other person.

One of the main problems with the transmission of sexually transmitted disease is that about 80% of people who are infected with any of these diseases have absolutely no symptoms from them. A person can have a sexually transmitted disease and not know of the infection. If asked by a potential sex partner about a sexually transmitted disease, those people can honestly say that they do not think they have one. Yet, they can have a germ which can be passed to that other person.

A very significant factor in this issue is that surveys show over and over that if a person is involved in a sexual lifestyle, they will lie to a potential sexual partner. S. D. Cochran reported that in a survey of sexually active college students many admitted lying in order to have sex. The lies included telling the other person that they had had fewer sexual partners than they had really had. Many of them said that even if they were involved with someone sexually they would not tell if they were having sex with another person at the same time.[26] It is this type of deception which allows many people to spread sexually transmitted disease to another person.

Is the solution to teach the traditional safe-sex message in a more aggressive way? I would propose that if a technique is not working, to re-double efforts with the same technique will not make it more effective. In one of the most condemning articles which has been written about traditional safe sex, J. W. Stout said "Five studies were identified in which the effects of sex education on these outcomes were evaluated. The available evidence indicates that there is little or no effect from school-based sex education on sexual activity, contraception or teenage pregnancy."[27]

Over and over we see statements such as, "The failure of such general education is particularly discouraging." This statement was made by T. M. Vernon in *The Journal of the American Medical Association* in his discussion of sex education.[28]

We have spent more than $3 billion in the U.S. on sex education programs. The level of sexual activity, the number of teenage pregnancies, and the abortion rate all have gone up almost with direct correlation to the increased amount of money spent on the traditional sex education programs we have been using. These sex education programs seem in some way to be causing young people to increase their sexual activity if the amount of money and its correlation to increased sexual activity can be used as an indicator.

Teach Abstinence Now

Some would say it is naive to believe that teenagers will hear that they should be abstinent until marriage and follow that guideline. Studies show, though, that this is a message that teenagers will hear. Examples are:

IN SCHOOLS—Teen Aid Abstinence Program

> *San Marcos High School - California*
> *The year before the program—*
> *147 pregnancies in 600 girls*
> *The year after —20 pregnancies*

> *Spur, Texas*
> *The year before—*
> *11 pregnancies in 450 girls*
> *The year after —1 pregnancy*

These results are from two high schools. Some would say this type of program might work in a high school but not in a community. In answer to that I mention an astounding study done at Grady Memorial Hospital in Atlanta. In this study conducted by Emory University Medical School, low-income teens were taught the value of delaying sexual intercourse. The results of this study showed that students who had not been in the program were five times more likely to have started having sex than the ones who had participated in the program.

It is quite obvious that if schools and parents and churches teach kids that they should be abstinent until they get married, they will hear this message. It is important that people who teach this message be enthusiastic about it. They should not be afraid to be directive. If they tell a student that as soon as they feel mature and responsible they can make a decision about sex, young people assume that it is okay for them to have sex and will frequently choose to do so because they feel they have the blessing of those people who are teaching them. It is important, therefore, that teachers and parents be directive to kids and tell them that they should not have sex until they get married, just as teachers and parents are now telling kids they should not smoke and should not use drugs.

It is important for parents and teachers to be honest with students and let them know that condoms will not protect them from sexually transmitted disease and that, indeed, they have an almost 20% chance of producing a pregnancy, even if they are using birth control pills for contraception.

Many of our young people have had intercourse. We can encourage them to avoid intercourse if their present sexual relationship breaks up. We need to show them that the more sexual partners they have, the more likely they are to get a sexually transmitted disease. They can stop having sex now, not have sex again until they get married, and avoid many of the problems they might have in their future if they continue relating to a person of the opposite sex with sexual intercourse.

Those of us who were of reproductive age prior to 1960 know that it is normal for an individual to reserve sexual intercourse until marriage because most people prior to 1960 did that. It has been the "sexual convulsion" of the past thirty years which has shown us that sex outside of marriage and that a great amount of sexual mixing with people going from one partner to another produces disease that not only makes people infertile but also kills them. The following points about abstinence are significant:

It was the norm prior to the sexual convulsion of the past thirty years.

It fits what we have learned in drugs and cigarette education.

It gives adolescents an expected standard to live up to.

It is the only solution.

It works!

Endnotes

[1]Spivak, H., Weitzman, *JAMA*, vol. 258, 18 September 1987, 1500-1504.

[2]This was reported by H. L. Brown, et al., *Southern Medical Journal*, 84:46, (1991).

[3]*The Perinatal Advocate* reported in 1991.

[4]In its *Morbidity and Mortality Weekly Report* , vol. 39, nos. 51 & 52 (4 January 1991).

[5]H. Bower, et al., *JAMA*, 23 January 1991, No. 4, 472-477.

[6]*Chlamydia Infections,* published by The American College of OB/GYN, 1987.

[7]H. Bower, et al., *JAMA*, 265:472, 1991.

[8]J. Apuzzio, *Medical Aspects of Human Sexuality*, (February 1990): 15 and Centers for Disease Control, 1991.

[9]Verbal communication from CDC, 1991; *Austin American Statesman*, 14 July 1991.

[10]CDC statistics.

[11]CDC, 1991—verbal communication.

[12]CDC statistics.

[13]CDC statistics.

[14]A. E. Washington, et al, *Journal of Adolescent Health Care*, (July 1985): 298.

[15]W. D. Mosher, et al., *Sexually Transmitted Disease,* 12 (1985):117.

[16]This problem was pointed out very clearly by J. Martinez, et al, in *Pediatrics,* 82 (1988):604.

[17]In *Family Planning Perspectives,* 23 (1991): 134-138.

[18]American College of Obstetricians and Gynecologists Newsletter, (March 1991):3.

[19]*OB/GYN Diagnosis,* Vol. 6, No. 3, (1987): 7.

[20]Reported in *Pediatric News* (May, 1990): 14.

[21]*The New England Journal of Medicine* , Vol. 322: 821.

[22]Margaret A. Fischl, M.D., et al., *Journal of the American Medical Association*, Vol. 257, No. 5, (6 February 1987): 640.

[23]S. Samuels, *Medical Aspects of Human Sexuality*, Vol. 23, (December 1989): 16.

[24]Ibid.

[25]Dr. Minkoff, *OB/GYN Audio Digest*, Vol. 37, No. 20, (1990).

[26]S. D. Cochran, *The New England Journal of Medicine*, Vol. 322, (March 1990): 774.

[27]J. W. Stout, *Pediatrics,* 83 (1989): 375-379.

[28]T. M. Vernon, *The Journal of the American Medical Association*, Vol. 260, No. 22, (9 December 1988).

Bioethics in the Third Millennium

By Nigel M. de S. Cameron

A combination of material prosperity and the seeming slowness of ethical change has helped cushion Christians from seriously reflecting upon what is taking place in our own society. For example, the covenantal family has collapsed as the normative unit of social life; and the interesting, if increasingly depressing, question is whether it will even survive as the norm for mainstream evangelicals.

We find ourselves in a generation that is bridging two different societies, one which was essentially continuous with Christendom and the other which is radical and untried in its pluralist sense of identity and which promises to be open to anything except the Christian religion it has finally succeeded in sloughing off. It is ironic that in the United States the secularization of the media and of public life—and, of course, particularly of public education—should have proceeded further and faster than in Europe, despite church attendance rates ten times as high. At this unique point in history, Christian young people are stepping out into a situation of profound cultural hostility, in which at every level they are challenged to conform to the increasingly settled assumptions of a post-Christian society. This is true, of course, and tragically so, in their marriages. It is even true in their assumptions about church membership. And it is focused sharply in their vocational commitment.

Of this there is no better example than medicine, for a number of reasons. For one thing, despite its pagan roots, the western medical tradition has been suffused by Christian values. Medicine continues to play a leading role in the determination of what constitutes a profession: as goes medicine goes the professional idea, in self-discipline, in the bundling of values and techniques, in the distinguishing of compensation from mere fee-for-service contractualism, and so forth. The special role of medicine derives, of course, in part from its unique place in human experience, as it deals with those moments when our humanity is laid bare in its tenuous hold on health and happiness, at birth and death, and in sickness and pain.

Medicine is handed down to us as an exercise constituted by moral commitments. To be precise, there are certain highly specific ethical requirements, and, as their context, a general characterization of the profession as a moral enterprise. That is the legacy of the early marriage of Hippocratic paganism with the Judeo-Christian tradition. If we look around us at the cultural benefits which we have all inherited from the Christendom centuries, we might consider our humane medical tradition as the jewel in the crown. As a result, what happens to medicine is fraught with special significance for our society and its values. And while this account is highly colored, there is wide recognition of the social significance of the break-up of the old certainties in medical values, both in the bifurcation of value and technique, and in the shift in substantive conviction on particular questions.

Recognition in the wider community has issued in the development of the discipline of bioethics. It stands at the interface of a series of disciplines—including medicine, but also law, biology, philosophy, theology—with vital connections to public policy discussion at every level. Among evangelicals, the only significant response has been engagement in the pro-life movement, almost as an article of faith, offering political and also practical focus to its deep unhappiness with the move to liberal abortion. These two responses—the pro-life movement and the burgeoning of academic bioethics—have had almost no connection, in that the bioethics establishment is generally contemptuous of the pro-life movement, while the pro-life movement has spawned remarkably little serious discussion of the questions back of the abortion debate. Moreover, in a country uniquely rich in evangelical educational plants, the resources presently committed to bioethics—which in secular academia has proved an area of quite phenomenal growth, measured by the usual indices: journals, institutes, programs, conferences, and finally jobs—are perplexingly small.[1]

But what *is* happening to medicine? As we move toward the third millennium, where is it going? Let me offer you a perspective. If we would avoid myopia, we must see liberal abortion not as a disease, but rather as a symptom of altogether broader distress within our medical culture. Antipathy toward abortion is one of the planks of a medical tradition which goes back more than two thousand years, with its origins in the kind of medicine being practiced by the disciples of Hippocrates of Cos. Though he was the most distinguished clinician of antiquity, Hippocrates' life is shrouded in uncertainty, as is his precise relation to the famous Oath and the many other writings associated with his name. What is plain is that a highly distinctive way of practicing medicine emerged in the Greece of late antiquity, characterized both by an understanding of medicine as an irreducibly moral exercise, and by a set of specific principles according to which (and *only* according to which) the Hippocratic physician would practice his art. However it originated, the Oath both offers a summary of those principles and sets them in a special context: That is to say, the Oath is an oath; the grounding of Hippocratic medical values is overtly theistic. While the theism was originally that of (probably Pythagorean) paganism, the values, their theistic grounding, and the vision they offered of medicine as an essentially moral enterprise commended them to the first Christians. The western tradition of Christian Hippocratism has been transmitted right down to the last portion of the twentieth century almost intact. What is symbolized in the reversal of two millennia of medical opposition to abortion is the beginning of the end of that tradition, the unraveling of its seamless dress.[2]

I have already made reference to the unremarkable fact that the Hippocratic Oath is an oath. The implications of this peculiar packaging of medical values have been little noted. It sets medicine in a context of covenant: a covenant of the physician with God, of the physician with the patient, of the physician with the profession. It is this three-fold covenant which holds in place the uniquely humane medical vision to which both doctor and patient are committed by the specific injunctions of the Oath. Unlike every modern re-write, the Oath is no mere moral code, but a lively exercise in theological ethics.

The injunctions, of course, are well-known: no abortion; no physician-assisted suicide (and since that term is now in vogue as a kind of best-case version of euthanasia, it is worth pointing out that it is specifically condemned in the Oath); no exploitation of the consulting situation—so we find a high doctrine of confidentiality (even including what the doctor picks up outside his professional relationship with the patient); a ban on sexual contacts, not just with the patient but even with the patient's slaves; and a general refusal to act in any way against the interests (though not necessarily the wishes) of the patient. It was such a packaging of skills and values that declared medicine a profession—indeed, had much to contribute to the development of the idea of a profession, as something other than a mere contractual exercise in fee-for-service. The disintegration of the professional character of medicine is not the least alarming feature of the post-Hippocratic situation.

The contrast is stark. In the place of the Hippocratic blending of values and skills, the notion of medicine as technique is almost *de rigueur* in a self-consciously pluralist society; yet its novelty within the western tradition is hardly acknowledged. At the same time, the central substantive moral commitment of the tradition has been discarded: the sanctity of human life, the major premise of the twin Hippocratic repudiations of abortion and suicide/euthanasia. The new discipline of bioethics has been generated to devise an alternative model of the medical enterprise in which, supposedly, patient autonomy serves in the place of covenantal Hippocratism in governing the moral relations of physician and patient. That is one reason why bioethics has become so much concerned to address questions of procedure, and so little interested in the old substantive issues of ethics. Who is to decide between prolife and pro-abortion? The imperative is to be pro-choice. The major task of bioethics has lain in devising the protocols of a pluralist medical culture.

The problem is that however *necessary* such an exercise may seem to be, it has little beyond seeming necessity to argue its potential for success. In repudiating consensus Hippocratism, we are placing the full weight for ethical choices in medicine upon the patient. Surprise, surprise: The typical patient is in rather a poor state to be making fundamental moral choices, especially if we happen to be persuaded that in order to be truly moral they require to be adequately informed. Aside perhaps from the retired medical professor who has taken up bioethics in his dotage, who is sufficient for these things? There is growing evidence in the literature to support our expectation that, for example, patients are very

heavily influenced in their choices by the spoken or unspoken pref-
erences of their physicians and their families. The sudden appearance of euthanasia on the western scene after so many centuries—
in Holland it is now common, if nominally still illegal, and in the
guise of physician-assisted suicide it will soon pass its first state
ballot here in the U.S.—focuses this question acutely. The notion
of the chronic or terminally sick, often depressed, anxious for their
family, frightened of dying, typically seeking to second-guess relatives who they think would be better off with them dead—the
notion of patients in such situations giving anything approaching
a "freely informed consent" to be killed would be ridiculous were it
not quite so disturbing.

Part of the special problematic of our situation arises from the
infusion of an array of fresh technological possibilities into traditional clinical and ethical situations. By tragic coincidence they are
posing us fateful questions at a time when we are less able than
for many hundreds of years to offer coherent answers. Abortion
and suicide/euthanasia, of course, are as old as sinful human society. Such options as *in vitro* fertilization, germline gene therapy,
and the bewildering range of life-preserving possibilities that we
associate with tubes and plugs at the intensive-care bedside are
new to our generation; yet the choices they offer us we are less and
less able to make, as the consensus in medical values goes into
free-fall. The radical privatizing of these choices in a kind of con-
sumerist ethics holds much attraction, and ultimately offers the
sole alternative to consensus, if consensus is regarded as unattain-
able or unattractive or both. Yet if the significance of these acts of
moral choice is so questionable (and it is interesting to ask even
bioethicists how they coped with real-life treatment decisions as
patients), we must ask what is actually happening behind the necessary smoke screen of the atomized medical culture of patient
autonomy? Plainly, the language of autonomous choice is serving—despite the best of intentions on the part of so many
involved—as cover for a developing, manipulative medicine, in
which behind the smoke the interests of other parties (insurers,
government, relatives, doctors, hospitals) are asserting themselves, overtly or otherwise, to determine the outcome of supposedly patient choices. That is why the move to some kind of euthanasia regime is so threatening, for then that ultimate choice for
death is subject to just the same kind of pressures, yet behind a
facade of respect for the patient's autonomy.

Of course, the bioethics agenda is long, and gets longer every
day. There are many options already accessible or just around the

corner which present dramatic challenges to our ethical insight and our power to control what takes place. We have already in small measure embarked on the harvesting of fetal organs and other tissue. If the dignity of the fetus is such that liberal abortion has become seemingly unchallengeable, it is hard to see us long holding out against the medical-commercial exploitation of the fetus in a comprehensive manner. The breeding of fetal humans to serve as donor banks for transplant and other programs may be hard to imagine in current circumstances, yet would represent merely one kind of resolution of the present legal and moral ambiguity in which fetal life is held.

A related development would bring to term the long-delayed development of an artificial placenta, in order that *in vitro* embryos might be brought to viability without ever seeing the inside of a human uterus. Alternatively, of course, they could be used as donor banks or subjects for vivisection. Since the principle of deleterious experimental use of the early embryo has already been widely sanctioned, it is hard to see how such later use (which would certainly be filled with beneficial fruit for experimenters, transplant recipients, and others beside) will be able to be stopped, once development through to the fetal stage *in vitro* is a possibility. No one doubts that it is a mere matter of technological progress until such possibility becomes actual.

We are already beginning to see advantage being taken of the many possibilities for managing death and manipulating both its time and its manner. We are certainly entering a period of human history when the management of death in western societies will be a cultural benchmark, seeming to set aside old taboos with a new can-do manipulativism. Though heralded as the triumph of human autonomy over the final barrier to its exercise, we will rapidly see the erosion of the voluntary requirement—as already in Holland, where the future has arrived. And, we must keep noting, euthanasia considered as billable medical procedure (a kind of anti-medicine) is remarkably cheap.

Exploration of the human genome holds extraordinary opportunities for good and evil, as we gain access to a new world of power over ourselves, for use and abuse. If the use fallen humankind has made of other technologies is a guide, we have cause to be alarmed; the possibilities for abuse will here be uniquely destructive of human dignity. Whether the current disinclination to favor germline interventions will long outlast the possibility of serious seeming benefit from such process remains to be seen. The marrying of advantage to patient and physician-scientist alike with the rhetoric of autonomy and choice may prove unstoppable.

Among these disturbing scenarios there are, of course, real problems to be addressed, and the challenge is to handle them responsibly and to maintain what the late Paul Ramsey called the hallmark of moral seriousness—the ability to say that there are some things we will never do. Yet that is not the hallmark of contemporary bioethical discussion, either cloistered in the academy or in the corridors of power as policy is written. Indeed, the contemporary bioethics community has generally worked within a remarkably secular and humanistic framework, and its first principle has been the repudiation of the Judeo-Christian and Hippocratic tradition, and its general supplanting by pluralist models which typically hinge on ideas of autonomy.

Practical Conclusions

The reason we survey the future is to prepare ourselves and our community—evangelical Christians in happy collaboration with others who will join with us–for a wholly different quality of understanding of these questions. We may speculate on the kind of issues that will face us and our children in ten, twenty, thirty years' time, but we cannot be sure. We must put ourselves in the best possible position to anticipate technological possibilities, society's response in both general social attitude and the formulation of public policy, and how we shall position ourselves as the church of Jesus Christ in the ensuing situation. How shall we conduct ourselves? How shall we lead and counsel our Christian people? How shall those in professional roles respond? What will be our own contribution to the policy debate—in the pulpit, in our schools, on picket lines, in academic journals, on Capitol Hill?

We must prepare, for time—too much time—has been lost. Quoting the prophet, Winston Churchill wrote of the lost years of the 1930s, when the democracies should have been re-arming and preparing to face the Nazis, as the locust years. For twenty years and more, the rise of the new bioethics has been a major phenomenon in academic and policy discussion. Save on the one issue of abortion, we have hardly had anything to say.

1. We must develop creative programs in church education. The conference at which these papers were given was a rarity. We must educate believers so they have a firm grasp of the implications—personal, professional, policy—of these seemingly arcane discussions.

2. To that end, we must make much better use of our theological seminaries to help our pastors lead the thinking of those whom they teach. I get calls from pastors who are perplexed in the face of these challenges—*in vitro*, genetic counseling and testing situations, the living will option—and they have no inkling of how to respond.

Of course, theological seminaries are always being blamed for something, and always being asked to do something else. But if these questions are half as significant as many of us believe, we must act.

3. Moreover, this nation is uniquely rich in its wealth of Christian investment in higher education; and our Christian colleges must rise to the challenge of preparing nurses and physicians and administrators as well as the other professionals for whom these issues are of special significance, and who need to gain crucial orientation during their time in college. Yet the responsibility is widely shirked. Pre-med and nursing programs may include no formal ethics component at all, or (as in a leading Christian college) it may be merely an elective. That is a devastating indictment of the failure of the evangelical community to wake up to the wider context of abortion.

That must be turned around, and our Christian colleges enabled to take a lead in offering an alternative education to our children, in which Christian distinctives form the context of the whole, and not merely an adjunct. In particular, we have it within our power to prepare a radically different kind of physician, who consciously places him or herself in the Christian-Hippocratic tradition. That will not happen unless we take bioethics much more seriously in Christian higher education.

4. Behind the teaching in our colleges and seminaries, back of our lobbyists and policy groups, and our church education projects, we desperately need a reflective research community of evangelicals on the leading edge of bioethics discussion—to bring together interdisciplinary consultations at the highest levels, to monitor the bioethics community worldwide so we have the best information, to develop international collaboration. There are many centers and institutes in the bioethics mainstream. As we face the future we must pray for that kind of provision for ourselves.

And we must do so facing the fact that, as the Lord tarries, the future seems to belong to the "New Medicine": post-consensus, post-Hippocratic, feeding on an illusory model of autonomy which seems to be demanded by the self-consciously pluralist character of the post-Christendom society; offering cover for a developing manipulative medical culture in which patients are finally subservient to the "interests" of an assortment of other parties. At the same time, there has been a staged withdrawal from the twin substantive values of Hippocratism—the sanctity of life and the principle of service we know as Hippocratic philanthropism.

The pagan foundations of the Hippocratic tradition, and the central place of humane medicine in western culture, make it peculiarly fertile ground for the development of a Christian alternative, not as a monastic exercise in withdrawal but as a declaration that there is a better way. We must call the profession back to its own highest goods and best self. There is some encouragement in the original context of the Hippocratic Oath and its bold, humane, alternative medicine. It began as the medical creed—the "manifesto," as it has been called—of a determined minority, intent upon the reformation of a medical culture in which doctors sat light to ethics and both abortion and euthanasia were accepted clinical options. We are called to dissidence, and a dauntless prophetic role in denunciation of evil and the pointing of a better way. The challenge to Christians is plain, and by the grace of God we shall rise to meet it.

Endnotes

[1] So the development of M.Div. and, especially, M.A. emphases at Trinity Evangelical Divinity School, which in a mainstream institution would be mere bandwagon jumping, takes on the appearance of serious innovation.

[2] This argument is traced at greater length in *The New Medicine*, Crossway, 1992.

PART V
Summary and Conclusion

Life at Risk:
We Must Not Fail

By Richard D. Land

It is a delight to deal with issues that are of such absolutely critical importance at an absolutely critically important time in the history of our nation and in the history of Western civilization.

In Deuteronomy 30:15-19, God's people were given a choice from God's messenger, sent by God Himself.

See, I have set before thee this day life and good, and death and evil; In that I command thee this day to love the Lord thy God, to walk in his ways, and to keep his commandments and his statutes and his judgments, that thou mayest live and multiply: and the Lord thy God shall bless thee in the land whither thou goest to possess it. But if thine heart turn away, so that thou wilt not hear, but shalt be drawn away, and worship other gods, and serve them; I denounce unto you this day, that ye shall surely perish, and that ye shall not prolong your days upon the land, whither thou passest over Jordan to go to possess it. I call heaven and earth to record this day against you, that I have set before you life and death, blessing and cursing: therefore choose life, that both thou and thy seed may live.

Every generation of God's people faces the same decision God placed before His people as they prepared to cross over Jordan and enter the Promised Land. Will they choose "life and good" or "death and evil," life and "blessing" or death and "cursing."

For more than a generation now, we as a people and as a nation have been discussing and debating the issues of life and death, what "life" means and whether or not it is "sacred."

The phrase, "sanctity of human life," encompasses a host of issues—abortion, infanticide, mercy-killing, "assisted" suicide, genetic engineering, fetal tissue experimentation—that have impacted, or will impact the life of every American. To believe in human life's sanctity is to understand that God created human beings "in his own image" (Gen. 1:26), the presupposition upon which the biblical doctrine of human life is based, thus imparting to them a special sanctity, unique among all created life.

While Genesis clearly identifies human beings as part of the created order, the emphasis is always on a uniqueness which is derived from human beings being made in God's image. That divine image, the *imago Dei*, which made relationship with God possible, was marred, but not obliterated by man's fall. God communicated with Adam and Eve both before (Gen. 1:28) and after (Gen. 3:9 ff.) the fall.

Psalm 8 juxtaposes man's limitations with his privileges and responsibilities, even as fallen creatures in a fallen world. Human beings, created "a little lower than the heavenly beings," are still "crowned with glory and honor" (Ps. 8:5, NIV) and given "dominion" over the rest of creation.

Even after the Fall, "the breath of the Almighty giveth them understanding" (Job 32:8, "understanding" being the Hebrew *binah,* meaning "discernment or wisdom"). Consequently, God tells fallen, but regenerate humanity, "Be ye not as the horse, or as the mule, which have no understanding" (Ps. 32:9), but instead that He would "instruct . . . and teach thee in the way which thou shalt go" (Ps. 32:8).

The central truth that emerges from these and other passages is that human life—all human life—is sacred, thus distinct from all other created life. We are different in nature and design from all other life. The differences are of *kind,* not *degree.* We are not merely the most advanced life in the animal kingdom.

The fact that all human life is sacred has serious personal, spiritual, moral, ethical, medical, and legislative implications for all "life" issues.

Unquestionably the most controversial "life" issue facing America today is abortion. For more than a generation now, we as a people have been choosing not life and blessing but death and cursing when it comes to our unborn children. We have been sacrificing our children to the false gods of career, convenience, and material well-being; and the magnitude of the slaughter is horrendous.

For twenty years we have been aborting a baby every 20 seconds, 3 babies a minute, 180 babies an hour, 4,320 babies a day, approximately 1.6 million babies a year. We have aborted one-third of an entire generation of America's children.

We have chosen death and cursing, rather than life and blessing. In our killing of 1.6 million children every year, have we aborted the girl God sent to find the cure for cancer? Have we destroyed the boy that God sent to find a cure for AIDS? Have we snuffed out the life of that one that God had gifted and prepared to lead us safely through some future national or world crisis? Have we aborted the one God sent to be the world's next great evangelist and soul winner? The odds are one in three that we have done precisely that.

In terms of sheer numbers, we have aborted approximately 30 million American babies since 1973. The oldest of these babies would now be in their second year of college or in the work force with a full lifetime of productivity before them. The economic and social costs of abortion are staggering and will seriously impact our ability to bear the medical and other retirement costs of the baby boom generation's elderly years. There are far too many in my generation who have aborted their babies in unprecedented numbers who, in our declining years, will be allowed or assisted to die before our natural time by our children and our grandchildren because they will consider us to be too expensive, too embarrassing, too ill, or too inconvenient. But as high as these costs are, the spiritual costs are even higher.

Abortion divides families, churches, communities, professional organizations, and political parties. And as terrible as it is, the killing of unborn babies is just the leading edge of the sanctity of life issue. The whole debate turns on whether human life is sacred or whether human beings are merely the most sophisticated life form in the animal kingdom.

If human life is sacred—and the Bible says that it is—then it is wrong to kill our unborn children because they have a *sacred* right to life which must not be denied. If one rejects human life's sanctity, however, and opts instead for a mere "quality of life" ethic, then you descend into a world in which unborn babies must meet certain parental criteria, such as being a wanted baby, a healthy baby, a "normal" baby, or an affordable baby, in order to be granted the *privilege* of life. Then you can kill, as we have done, millions of babies because their mothers considered them to be too embarrassing, too expensive, too ill, or too inconvenient to live outside the womb.

Let's make no mistake about it. We are talking about killing unborn babies. I have here a Letter to the Editor from the Nashville *Tennessean,* written by a mother.

Many people believe that abortion is acceptable in the early months of pregnancy because "it" wasn't a baby yet. I have recently had an experience that sheds some light on this subject.

I was 16 weeks pregnant when my doctor could not find a fetal heartbeat. An ultrasound confirmed that my baby had died. I chose to have labor induced and delivered a baby boy on February 5.

He weighed one ounce and was about four inches long. I held him in the palm of my hand! He had tiny hands and feet, his ears had formed, and I could count his ribs. He had died a week or two earlier, which puts him at around 12-14 weeks' gestation, which is still quite common for abortions.

[And under the proposed Freedom of Choice Act, this would be an unprotected child right up to the moment of birth by federal law.]

But this was a real baby! The hospital gave me footprints of my tiny baby. Can a "blob of tissue" have footprints? I am writing to testify that a "fetus" is a baby!

Something that shouldn't be a shock, since a fetus is described in all medical textbooks as a stage of human development.

If human life is sacred, it was inevitable from the beginning that it would become a womb-to-tomb debate. Human life is now under relentless assault in our culture, from conception to natural death and everywhere in between. The debate has moved to the nursery, where parents have now been granted the legal right by the United States Supreme Court in the *Baby Doe* case to allow their child to die because he was mentally handicapped. And so mental retardation becomes a death sentence.

The debate also now includes the nursing home and the intensive care unit. As we witness our courts defining the administration of food and water to unconscious patients as "extraordinary" medical means which may be withheld in certain circumstances, and as we hear on the evening news the controversy over mercy-killing and assisted-suicide, we see the consequences of the lethal quality-of-life ethic's assault on human life and its sanctity.

Will we allow fetal tissue experimentation on our unborn babies? Will we allow our society to encourage wholesale abortion in order to produce fetal tissue to harvest and use for whatever means they choose—medical, commercial, or cosmetic? As Ben Mitchell puts it in the Christian Life Commission's sanctity guide, "Will a mother's body become a human fetal tissue farm?" I, like most of you, was born into a society which revered human life. It was a society which condemned a social order (Nazism) which experimented on and harvested human beings for soap and lamp shades. Are we now destined to live out our lives in a society which denies human life's sanctity and condones the harvesting of fetal tissue and mercy-killing as well as wholesale abortion?

The Nazi death camps fifty years ago and the more recent Cambodian genocide illustrate what an alarmingly dangerous place the world is for those too young, too few, too old, too weak, too handicapped or too ill to defend their right to life when the sanctity of any human life is denied or denigrated.

Richard John Neuhaus, in a new book called *America Against Itself*,[1] speaks eloquently about the results of the *Cruzan* case where, for the first time, the courts of our land find the giving of food and water, hydration and nutrition, to a person who was in a persistent vegetative state as an extraordinary medical means that could be denied.

Who won and who lost in the *Cruzan* case? Was it a civilized step toward 'death with dignity,' or a brutal turn, cloaked in the rhetoric of compassion, toward ridding ourselves of the burdensome among us? Certainly it was a radical turn from long-established moral principle. The official directive for Catholic health facilities declares: "The directly intended termination of any patient's life, even at his own request, is always morally wrong."

And Dr. Neuhaus points out, "There is nothing particularly Catholic in that claim. In Western medicine, that principle has been in place since Hippocrates in the fifth century B.C. It has often been violated, also in modern times—massively so under Nazism and Communism—but civilized people have adhered to it in principle. No longer."

We have crossed that Rubicon where the doctor who is an agent for life, who is sworn to do no harm, now removes a feeding tube from a person who will then starve to death; and the clear intent is that the patient will be killed by the action of the doctor.

"At the risk of entering," Dr. Neuhaus says,"upon a heavily mined field, we must ask whether we can speak about lives not worth living without remembering the phrase, *lebensunvertes Leben?* It means in German, lives unworthy of life." It was the slogan under which the Nazis exterminated tens of thousands of people because they were mentally handicapped, because they were physically handicapped, because they were terminally ill.

Dr. Neuhaus says, "Yes, I know that none of us are Nazis, and this is not Germany in the 1930s. This is America, and we are motivated by kindness and compassion. It cannot happen here. We would never do that kind of thing."

What if we are, in fact, doing not only that kind of thing, but that very thing, killing people, in the name of compassion and kindness? It is one thing to allow someone to die, but it is another thing to take positive measures that result in that person's death. We are on the edge of a terrible abyss.

Will it happen here? Is it happening here? Much depends on the faith community. We are the last line of defense against a rapid descent into an evil abyss of barbarism. Christians must sound the clarion call against all attitudes and actions which assault the sacredness of human life. We must bear witness by deed as well as by word that human life is a sacred, precious, irreplaceable gift from God. We must oppose the barbaric, lethal combination of technical expertise and spiritual ignorance which would deny human life's sanctity and abort or experiment on our unborn, harvest fetal tissue, allow death into the nursery for our mentally and physically handicapped infants, and encourage euthanasia in our hospitals and in our retirement homes.

We have a biblically, divinely appointed task. God told Isaiah, "I have set watchmen upon thy walls, O Jerusalem, which shall never hold their peace day nor night: ye that make mention of the Lord, keep not silence" (Isa. 62:6). Those watchmen are an oft-mentioned thing in Scripture. In Jeremiah 6 God returns to the watchmen analogy.

> They have healed also the hurt of the daughter of my people slightly, saying Peace, peace; when there is no peace.

False teachers, who come with false solutions.

> Were they ashamed when they had committed abomination? nay, they were not at all ashamed, neither could they blush: therefore they shall fall among them that fall: at the time that I visit them they shall be cast down, saith the

Lord. Thus saith the Lord, Stand ye in the ways, and see, and ask for the old paths, where is the good way, and walk therein, and ye shall find rest for your souls. But they said, We will not walk therein. Also I set watchmen over you, saying, Hearken to the sound of the trumpet. But they said, We will not hearken. Therefore hear, ye nations, and know, O congregation, what is among them. Hear, O earth: behold, I will bring evil upon this people, even the fruit of their thoughts, because they have not hearkened unto my words, nor to my law, but rejected it (Jer. 6:14-19).

And then in Ezekiel 3:1: ". . . eat this roll, and go and speak to the house of Israel." If we are going to be God's watchmen, then we must eat the Word of God. As Spurgeon put it, "To eat our way into the Scripture until our blood is bibline." And then we go, standing on God's truth that all human life is sacred, that God has a plan and a purpose for every human life.

And then, listen to what happens.

Son of man, all my words that I shall speak unto thee receive in thine heart, and hear with thine ears. And go, get thee to them of the captivity, . . . and tell them, Thus saith the Lord God; whether they will hear, or whether they will forbear (Ezek. 3:10-11).

And it came to pass . . . Son of man, I have made thee a watchman unto the house of Israel: therefore hear the word at my mouth, and give them warning from me. When I say unto the wicked, Thou shalt surely die; and thou givest him not warning, nor speakest to warn the wicked from his wicked way, to save his life: the same wicked man shall die in his iniquity; but his blood will I require at thine hand. Yet if thou warn the wicked, and he turn not from his wickedness, nor from his wicked way, he shall die in his iniquity; but thou hast delivered thy soul (Ezek. 3:16-19).

We are called to be watchmen, whether they will hear or whether they will forbear, whether they will turn or whether they will not turn. God has given us our marching orders. And my prayer for each of us is to call Him Lord and that we, like the apostle Paul in taking his leave of the Ephesian elders, can say, "I am innocent of the blood of all men. I have not hesitated to proclaim all of God's truth" (Acts 20:26b-27).

It is, in the providence of God, our lot to live in a time when we are seeing the downward degradation and spiral of sin enunciated in Romans 1 lived out before our very eyes. And to have President Clinton, one who speaks our language, proclaims our truths, to say as he said on January 23, 1993, in *The New York Times,* having picked the twentieth anniversary of *Roe v. Wade* to sign the removal of the decrees of the previous administration: "We must let medicine and science proceed unencumbered by anti-abortion politics. We must free science and medicine from the grasp of politics and give all Americans access to the very latest and best medical treatments." The very latest and best medical treatments—I guess my first question there would be, "The very latest and best medical treatments for whom?" Certainly not the latest and best medical treatments for the babies who die. Certainly not the latest and best medical treatments for the handicapped infants who are allowed to starve to death like Baby Doe. Certainly not the very latest and best medical treatments for Miss Cruzan, who starved to death in a hospital in the United States of America, one nation, under God.

What the President calls "anti-abortion politics" are simply nothing less than questions of whether we ought to ask whether something is right or something is wrong. Whether something should never be done or should always be done. Whether or not God has anything to say to us. Now there are those who would argue that, in light of the experience of the last dozen years or so, Christians ought to withdraw from the public arena and concentrate on a moral reformation. That is a false dichotomy. It is an invention of the devil to say we should either be involved with winning souls and converting minds or we should be involved in politics. It is always required that we do both. Anyone who thinks that we were not concerned and will not be concerned about changing the hearts and the minds of men hasn't listened to what we've said. Perhaps they have just been reading and even rolling up and smoking some of the press releases that are written about us.

It is never enough to do one or the other. The transforming moral and cultural event of my life is a classic example of that. It was not enough to change the hearts and the minds of men and women in this country. We had to eradicate the blight of segregation on our land. It could not be done without changing hearts and minds, but it also could not be done without changing evil law. We must do both.

The watchman is given another reminder in Psalm 127:1: "Except the Lord build the house, they labour in vain that build it: except the Lord keep the city, the watchman waketh but in vain." Everything depends on God's blessings.

When in doubt, always go to Spurgeon. Here's a quote from Benjamin Franklin [Benjamin Franklin: Speech in Convention for

285

forming a Constitution for the United States, 1787] which is in Spurgeon's commentary on Psalm 127 (*The Treasury of David*, Vol. VII. p. 33):

In the beginning of the contest with Britain, when we were sensible of danger, we had daily prayers in this room for the Divine protection. Our prayers, sir, were heard, and they were graciously answered. All of us who were engaged in the struggle must have observed frequent instances of a superintending Providence in our favour. To that kind Providence we owe this happy opportunity of consulting in peace on the means of establishing our future national felicity. [This was at the time of the Constitutional Convention.] And have we now forgotten this powerful Friend? or do we imagine we no longer need his assistance? I have lived for a long time [81 years]; and the longer I live the more convincing proofs I see of this truth, that God governs in the affairs of man. And if a sparrow cannot fall to the ground without his notice, is it probable that an empire can rise without his aid? We have been assured, sir, in the sacred writings, that "Except the Lord build the house, they labour in vain that build it." I firmly believe this; and I also believe that without his concurring aid we shall proceed in this political building no better than the builders of Babel: we shall be divided by our little, partial, local interest; our prospects will be confounded; and we ourselves shall become a reproach and a by-word down to future ages. And what is worse, mankind may hereafter, from this unfortunate instance, despair of establishing government by human wisdom, and leave it to chance, war, or conquest. I therefore beg leave to move that henceforth prayers, imploring the assistance of Heaven and its blessing on our deliberations, be held in this assembly every morning before we proceed to business.

"Except the Lord build the house, . . . the watchman waketh but in vain." Make no mistake about it. It was never either/or. It is always both/and, a moral and spiritual reformation which results in laws that are pleasing to God. They are like the two blades of a pair of scissors. By themselves they are not much use, but together they can do what they were designed to do. And God designed the people of God to win the hearts and minds of people. And He designed government, in Romans 13, to punish those who do evil and to reward those who do that which is right. Make no mistake about it, the heart of man is deceitful and desperately wicked. If we didn't have laws against slavery, some people would own slaves. If we hadn't eradicated "Jim Crow," he would still be with us. We did it, not by the force of law alone and not by moral reformation alone, but by the two working together in divine Providence.

I pray that our Heavenly Father will use all of us to contend with diligence and discernment for the sanctity of human life. My prayer is that we will remember that the "watchman waketh but in vain" unless God blesses. I pray that we will stride forth in God's strength and with God's blessing to help our nation rebuild the walls with a sword and a trowel and complete the journey back to a civilized society founded on the Judeo-Christian moral values which honor and protect human life's sanctity.

If we fail to insist that our society be one in which it is always wrong to do certain things to a human being, then we are bound to live in a society in which virtually anything can, and will, be done to human beings.

Endnotes

[1]Richard John Neuhaus, America Against Itself: Moral Vision and the Public Order, (Notre Dame, Ind.: University of Notre Dame Press, 1992).